# STROKE OF LOVE

## MEMOIR OF
## NANCY SPANO

Copyright © 2024 | Stroke of Love Publishing

Nancy Spano
spanonancy@gmail.com

ISBN: 979-8-9901362-0-5
Edition: First Edition
Version: First print version

EDITOR: David Lloyd Strauss
INTERIOR DESIGN: Hmdpublishing
COVER LAYOUT: Hmdpublishing

PROFILE PHOTO LICENSED BY:
Marty Umans Photography
426 Blinn Rd
Croton on Hudson, NY 10520
MartyUmans.com

All rights reserved. No part of this publication may be reproduced, distributed, or transmitted in any form or by any means, including photocopying, recording, or other electronic or mechanical methods, without the prior written permission of the publisher, except in the case of brief quotations embodied in critical reviews and certain other non-commercial uses permitted by copyright law. For permission requests, reach out through davidstrauss.com.

All animated images were created with Dall-E using custom prompts.

ORDERING INFORMATION:
Special discounts are available on quantity purchases by corporations, associations, and organizations. Contact the publisher at the above address for special discounts.

SERIES: STROKE OF LOVE SERIES

# DEDICATION

*If not for my husband and best friend, none of this would be possible. He has not only supported me financially, but he has also stood by me through thick and thin, for better or worse. Because of his support, I'm able to continue to increase my momentum to be the best speaker and author.*

*To my beautiful daughters, Ava and Abigail, you are my dream come true and the strength behind my will to survive and thrive.*

*And to all those navigating the turbulent waters of illness and disease, may this book serve as a testament to the resilience of the human spirit. Remember, within you lies an indomitable force capable of overcoming the greatest challenges. May you find the courage to persevere, the strength to endure, and the hope to envision a future filled with brighter days.*

# FOREWORD

Nancy Spano's "Stroke of Love" is a journey through life's ups and downs, a true story of overcoming adversity with grace, a little bit of grit and whole lot of determination. Nancy invites us into her world with the warmth of a friend as she shares all the mental, physical, and emotional moments which led to her mind, body and spiritual healing.

"Stroke of Love" is more than a book, it's a heartfelt guide to finding light in the darkness, strength in vulnerability, and triumph in the face of seemingly insurmountable obstacles.

So, as you dive into Nancy's world, be prepared to laugh, cry, and ultimately, feel inspired. This isn't just Nancy's story; it's a mirror reflecting our own potential to navigate life's challenges with resilience and love.

**Stephanie Arnold**
Writer. Producer. Speaker. Thought Leader.

# PROLOGUE

"Stroke of Love" is my heartfelt response to God's call, an invitation to share my journey through the valleys of depression, the shadows of childhood trauma, and my battles against cancer and stroke. It's a story of vulnerability, resilience, and the power of faith.

Life presents us all with a series of obstacles and tests. My path has been strewn with hurdles, each an opportunity to rise stronger with God's grace. He gives His biggest battles to His strongest warriors; my life has been a testament to this belief. From the grip of depression rooted in childhood trauma to the profound loss of loved ones, my faith has been my beacon, guiding me through the darkest times.

The journey to reclaim my spirit involved deep introspection and an unwavering commitment to shift my perspective from victim to victor. "Stroke of Love" offers clarity and inspiration, empowering you to harness your inner strength and resilience in the face of life's trials. Every day, I'm thankful for the chance to rewrite my story and to inspire others to navigate their challenges with courage and hope.

Life is about those special moments that we never forget. The ones where we don't remember what happened beforehand or what happened afterward; we only remember that split second that changed our life. That was the moment for me. It was a ho-hum day, and I had installed a new app on my phone called Clubhouse. I was learning how to navigate it. There were live rooms with different titles and topics. I gravitated to a room that was discussing tools on how to overcome adversity. Some people chose to raise their hands and share their stories. At first, I laid low and listened to everyone else's share. Something stirred inside me, and I lifted my hand to speak. Suddenly, my adrenaline started to pump, and I felt empowered. Before I was done sharing my story, a voice interrupted and unmuted her microphone. She says, "Oh my goodness, when are you writing your book?".

I thought, book? What book? I'm not a writer; I don't have what it takes to be an author. I believe everyone has a story, and it's up to them whether to sit on the sidelines and miss out on the action or get in the game and help others along on their journey. One of my favorite verses from the Bible is, "FAITH the size of a mustard seed can move mountains." That split second was my mustard seed, and I continue to move mountains.

I didn't take any action with that statement for a while, but it continuously resonated in the back of my head. "When are you going to write your book?"

Well, until this next moment, I was sitting on the sidelines. It was about a year after that night in Clubhouse. I was resting with my youngest daughter. Around 3 a.m., I felt a nudge and heard a voice say, "Get up and write this down." I tossed and turned and tried to ignore it, but it was relentless. I heard again, "Get up and write this down, or you'll never forgive yourself." Ugh, I was so warm and comfortable, but I knew the sooner I listened, the sooner I could return to bed. I walked out of my daughter's room, through the dining room, into the kitchen. It was dark, and I didn't dare turn on the light. I grabbed anything that would write and some scrap paper. With my eyes closed, I wrote what He told me to write and hurried back to bed.

The next morning, as I entered the kitchen to make my coffee, I noticed the chicken scratch on the scrap paper. It said, "STROKE of LOVE," and that, folks, is how this dream became my reality.

# Contents


Introduction Embracing Life's Storms..............................11

01. Shadows of Uncertainty........................................15

02. The Day Normalcy Faded......................................25

03. Unraveling the Ties...............................................33

04. Finding My Voice................................................41

05. Journeys of Joy and Sorrow..................................55

06. Bittersweet Beginnings........................................63

07. Unraveling Shadows............................................75

08. Resilience in the Face of Adversity........................91

09. From Recovery to Revelation..............................103

10. Embracing Resilience.........................................111

Thank you..............................................................115

Acknowledgements.................................................119

About the Author....................................................123

Connect with Nancy...............................................125

# INTRODUCTION
# EMBRACING LIFE'S STORMS

## Thriving Through Struggle

~❖~
*"The great art of life is sensation;*
*to feel that we exist, even in pain."*
**—Lord Byron**
~❖~

Have you ever felt like life's relentless storms were tailor-made for you? As if every challenge and every setback were a personal test of your strength and resilience? Well, you're not alone. My story might echo yours in ways you never imagined. This isn't just a recollection of my battles; it's a mirror reflecting the universal struggle we all face in our unique ways.

I'm Nancy, and this book is more than just a chronicle of my life's toughest challenges. It's a journey we embark on together, exploring how adversity shapes us and how it's an integral part of our own stories of self-acceptance and growth. It's a tale that resonates with anyone who's ever faced health scares, emotional upheavals, or those silent battles fought in the solitude of one's heart.

Each chapter of my life, from grappling with a stroke and cancer scare to the relentless battle against Stage 4 endometriosis, isn't just a personal narrative. It's a testament to our resilience, a showcase of the mental and emotional fortitude we all possess but sometimes forget about in the chaos of life. This book is about thriving amidst adversity, not just surviving it.

But it's not just my story. As you journey through these pages, you'll see reflections of your own struggles and victories. You'll find parts of yourself in my journey – in the small triumphs, the hard-fought battles, and the unwavering belief in the beauty of life, even when it seems bleakest.

This book delves deep into the mind-body connection, exploring how our physical health is intrinsically linked to our emotional well-being. It's about understanding that our battles aren't just physical but emotional, mental, and deeply personal.

It's a story of victory, not victimhood, transforming our circumstances into stepping stones for growth and emerging stronger. It's about finding hope in the face of despair, strength in vulnerability, and joy in the simplest things in life. It's about seeing your reflection in my story and realizing you're not alone.

You're a part of this narrative, too – a tale of resilience, of the human spirit's indomitable will to overcome. This book is a beacon of hope for anyone feeling lost in their struggles, a reminder that pain is universal, but so is the strength to conquer it.

As you read, you'll find yourself rooting for me, empathizing with my struggles, and finding inspiration in my resilience. It's a journey that will teach you the art of transforming pain into a force that propels you forward, of seeing your challenges not as obstacles but as opportunities for growth and self-discovery.

Join me in this movement of embracing our scars and turning them into our greatest strengths. It's a story that will inspire you to face life's storms not with fear but with the courage to thrive through them. Welcome to a journey of transformation, resilience, and hope. Welcome to a story that's as much yours as it is mine. Welcome to our shared journey of embracing life's storms and finding the strength to thrive.

# Chapter One

# Shadows of Uncertainty

## The day everything shifted

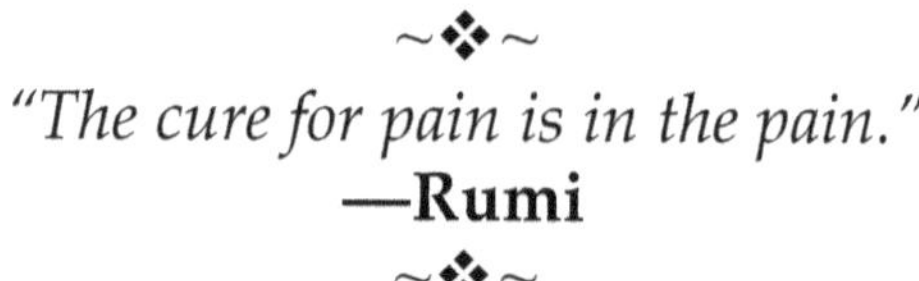

~❖~
*"The cure for pain is in the pain."*
**—Rumi**
~❖~

On May 25th, 2019, it started as a beautiful Saturday morning, or so I thought. My husband and I and our two girls piled into the car. We pulled out of our apartment complex parking lot and slowly made our way to the highway.

My family and I were preparing to drive an hour south of my home to visit my in-laws in White Plains, New York. When we were halfway there, I recall reclining my seat and feeling the sun coming in through the window, warming my face and the rest of my body. I was so warm and relaxed, like a cat on a windowsill.

At one point during the ride, I thought I felt my right arm go numb, but I brushed it off as nothing because I was so relaxed and warm. Everyone in the family was excited about the warm weather, the upcoming summer, and the opening of the pools in our area. We started early in the morning to squeeze every beautiful minute out of the day.

My mother-in-law always planned a Memorial Day celebration, and we were prepared to spend the holiday with them.

When we arrived at my in-laws', our family holiday went as planned. There was fruit, hamburgers, hotdogs, salad, and, of course, pasta. Every holiday, I was known for making my flag cake, a vanilla cake with cool whip, strawberries, and blueberries that acted as stars and stripes on the cake.

There was an energy amongst our family that day that couldn't be denied; everyone was happy. We were looking forward to what Nona, my husband's mother, had on the menu that day. She's originally from Italy, and her homemade cooking is to die for.

We all sat and enjoyed each other's company and, of course, dessert. It was getting dark, and we started to clean up and say our goodbyes. None of us looked forward to the drive home, but we all got to rest while my husband drove us home.

The following day, Sunday, started without a hitch. I could hear birds chirping outside my window and looked forward to another beautiful day. I made my bed as I talked to myself about the layout of the plans for the day. My mind usually races about what is on my daily agenda.

After making the bed and getting dressed, I headed downstairs for my first sip of sanity. My family knows to talk to me when I have that first cup of coffee.

As the day progressed, I noticed subtle changes in how I felt. Normally, my husband and I had a caring and loving relationship, but as we went about our day, I started feeling very irritable and short-tempered with everyone, especially my husband.

I have a history of Thyroid disease, which requires my blood levels to be adjusted quarterly. Sometimes, when my blood levels are not balanced properly or I'm overdue for a checkup, I feel exhausted, irritable, and short-tempered.

On the day that I could not get along with my husband, I thought this was the issue. There are several types of thyroid disease.

I have a history of Graves disease and was diagnosed around 25 years old. According to the Mayo Clinic, it is an autoimmune disease that leads to an overactive thyroid gland. This autoimmune disease is also known to mistakenly attack healthy tissue.

At age twenty-five, I developed a goiter in my neck, which means the thyroid glands are enlarged. Even though I believe everything happens for a reason, my thyroid disease was found by accident.

I was between jobs in 1998, so I had no health insurance. While unemployed, I went to a nearby Planned Parenthood, and I was examined. When I laid back on the table, the nurse looked at me in an odd way. I asked, "Is something wrong? Is everything OK?"

She said she was concerned about the size of my neck. She went on to state that I might have a goiter. I responded with a "What?" She explained that a goiter happens when your thyroid gland becomes enlarged. I knew my older brother suffered from thyroid disease, and I told her that I had been checked multiple times throughout the years. She said, "The blood test is not expensive, and if you are suffering from thyroid disease, it needs to be taken care of."

I agreed to the blood test, and then I went on my way home.

I recall my visit to Planned Parenthood being on a Friday because, on Monday morning, I received a frantic call from the nurse. She said, "Your thyroid levels are completely abnormal, and you need to see an endocrinologist as soon as possible." That experience was my first introduction to my uphill battle with thyroid disease.

Within weeks of being diagnosed with thyroid disease, I also learned I had a condition called Wolff-Parkinson-White syndrome (WPW). It means I was born with an extra electrical pathway to my heart. After the radioactive medication for my thyroid, I underwent a procedure where a catheter was inserted into my groin, and with every heartbeat, it climbed up to my heart. I watched the whole process on the monitor. Once the catheter reached my heart, my doctor went behind a curtain, like the Great Oz in The Wizard of Oz, and pressed a button. It delivered an enormous amount of heat to my chest, which I later learned was from when they were cauterizing the extra electrical pathway. Through my research, it is not uncommon for people who suffer from thyroid disease to also have health issues concerning their hearts.

I received radioactive treatment for it. The radioactive treatment comes in the form of a pill, and it is so powerful that it kills the thyroid gland, and the goiter disintegrates. The pill was given to me in capsule form. It was carefully placed in a ball made of concrete and administered to me. After ingesting the radioactive medication, I had to wait about 24-48 hours before I could be around anyone due to the radioactivity within the capsule. After the medication was ingested, hyperthyroidism became hypothyroidism, and I'm now on medication to regulate it for the rest of my life.

I tried my best to go about my day, but doing basic everyday activities became tough. My typical daily routine was to shower, dry off, and dry my hair. I picked up my hairdryer, held the cord in my hand, and continued to look at the plug on the wall. As I looked back at the cord and then the hairdryer, I couldn't figure out how to plug it in for the life of me.

Why was this happening suddenly, and what was going on with me? Daily activities are sometimes taken for granted until you cannot complete them alone.

I stood in the bathroom, feeling dazed and confused. What is happening? Am I just imagining this? I genuinely don't know what's going on.

It felt like my insides were constantly trembling with internal tremors. It was challenging to hold the cord steady and line it up correctly with the plug on the wall. It was frustrating because of what was happening inside my body. I didn't want anyone to think I was weird or crazy; no one knew about this issue but me. I attempted numerous times to plug the dryer in, but my fine motor skills kept holding me back.

Later, during the same week, my husband asked me to button his lapel, and I couldn't manage to get my fingers to work. I told him, "This is crazy; what's happening to me?" "Honey, my fine motor skills are screwed up, and I feel like my insides are constantly trembling!" My husband shrugged his shoulders and left because he was late for work. The next day, I realized that brushing my teeth was also tricky.

I never dreamed that a simple task like brushing my teeth could be so difficult. I couldn't hold my toothbrush steady enough to get my teeth clean. Putting the cap on the toothpaste was difficult; my internal tremors wouldn't let up enough to screw the cap on. I tried to keep pushing forward with my daily chores, but inside, I was struggling and confused. Every minuscule task became an obstacle. I became depressed, angry, and a little frightened.

It was coming toward the end of the week, and I usually drive my girls to school in the morning. We all woke up and got ready for school. The house was chaotic in the morning, so I didn't have time to notice anything unusual. I served the girls their breakfast, dressed them, and we went out the door. I settled the girls in their seats and started the car.

My parking spot is right alongside the big yellow curb, and I usually use it as a marker to pull out. I didn't put my seatbelt on yet, so I could twist my body to look out the back and passenger window to make sure I cleared the curb. Something was funny, but not in a humorous way. I sat back and realized there was something wrong with my right eye. I removed my glasses and looked at them to make sure I didn't smudge them with my fingers. I had just had an eye exam, and I was given a new prescription for my lenses. I thought maybe the doctor screwed up. Nothing was on my glasses, so I put them back on and continued to back up.

Again, I looked out of the passenger side window so I could use the big yellow curb as a marker to get out of my spot, but I couldn't see the curb. I've worn glasses for seven years, and I usually need them to read and for distance, so this lack of sight in one eye was unusual. I became nervous and unsettled, especially with my two young girls in the car, and I remember feeling uneasy about driving them around.

It took all my strength not to share my feelings of uneasiness with them, and inside I just wanted to cry.

I dropped them both off at school and hoped whatever was happening to me would go away. I attempted to go about my day but continued to have setbacks. The internal tremors continued and affected everything, from doing dishes to folding laundry. It felt as though someone had pulled a shade from my eye. I recall my mother speaking about patients experiencing a shade being pulled down on one eye in the past because she witnessed it in nursing, but I don't remember where she said it was from.

Realizing that I had lost the peripheral vision in my eye was so scary, and I didn't know what to make of any of it. I usually share things that happen in my life with my mom, but somehow, I felt deep down that these symptoms were severe, and I didn't want to know the truth. I was scared, felt alone with my symptoms, and questioned everything that was happening to me.

Towards the week's end, I felt very frustrated and exhausted. My husband and I have a long history of laughing and joking together, and during whatever this crap was, we were bickering and constantly nitpicking. If I could've unzipped myself out of my skin and run away, I would have.

My family and I usually have so much fun together, and we are constantly telling jokes, being sarcastic, and sometimes being inappropriate. We enjoy our humor and our time together. Our girls go everywhere with us, and we enjoy their company. During the summertime, we spend our days at a nearby lake or pool. On a weekend morning, we would get up early, pack our lunches, get a cooler ready, fill it with water and iced tea, and plan to spend the whole day at the lake.

My husband and I would sit by the water and watch the girls play with friends. They would go up and down the water slide and come out every now and then to have a snack. We would pack up and head home when they got waterlogged and looked like raisins. We loved our summer days together, and we would take walks around our apartment complex at night. When we weren't at the lake or pool, we spent time at the dog park with our border collie or shooting baskets in the hoops out back.

My girls have lots of friends in the complex, and they spend time riding their bikes or playing with Barbies on the front steps. On hot summer nights, we would visit a local ice cream store and eat outside on the picnic tables. I feel very fortunate and grateful for such a wonderful husband and two incredible girls; we are truly blessed. Going out to dinner at a nearby steakhouse is a treat, and during the summer months, we go as often as possible. The energy in our home is welcoming and inviting, and we laugh every day. We all respect and love each other, so when one of us is having a bad day and needs space, we give it to them.

Sunday morning came around, and the energy in the house was negative. It was a beautiful, hot day at the beginning of June. Typically, we would spend the day at the pool. That was the last thing on my mind this morning. I just wanted to be alone, and everyone felt it. If I didn't live there, I wouldn't have wanted to be there myself. I woke up and didn't want to be around anyone. I came downstairs for breakfast, and I had such an attitude. I tried to get through breakfast, but my insides were shaking, and I just wanted to scream. My husband and daughters constantly asked me, "What's wrong with you?" "Why are you acting so nasty?" I would get so upset and have no answer for them. What was I supposed to say? I didn't have any answers.

My husband took me aside and said," I don't know what's going on with you, but obviously, you need some time alone. I will spend the day with the girls, and you can go out alone." Part of me was happy, and the other part was upset that I was so irritable, and no one wanted to be around me. My husband and the girls got themselves ready and left for the day.

The house was completely empty, and I was alone. I was alone with my thoughts, alone with my fear and anxiety, and alone with this monster that was taking over my body and my senses. Sometimes you have to be careful what you ask for because, like they say, "You might get it," and I did! Now that I was alone and had nothing but time, what would I do with myself?? I looked around my home with a lump in my throat and thought, "What the hell should I do?" Many emotions came up for me, one of them being hopelessness. I tried to pick myself up and get my shit together. I thought, OK, maybe I'll clean up and vacuum; that will help me feel more organized and accomplished.

So, the dialogue started in my head: "Where's the vacuum?" What?? What do you mean, where's the vacuum?? UGH, if I could've kicked myself, I would have. I eventually located the vacuum and decided to sit down and remove all the hair from the bristles; the vacuum usually works better that way. I've done this numerous times, and it was like second nature. So, I sat down on the rug and flipped the vacuum over. I started to sweat and became overwhelmed with the task. It didn't help that I could only see out of one eye. I know the steps by heart, and when I couldn't remember how to do them, I came down hard on myself. I wanted to throw the vacuum across the room and run away. With my internal tremors still affecting me, I tried to compose myself as best I could.

The vacuum was an upright model with a metal plate on the bottom holding it together. Plastic screws had slits in them that I could usually open with a butter knife. I went to the kitchen to grab the knife and sat back down. OK, now I can do this. I kept repeating. I was all thumbs!!!! OMG!! What in the world is going on with me?? I couldn't hold the butter knife steady; I couldn't remember how to unscrew the vacuum plate, and I just wanted to cry!! There was no one to ask for help. I felt like a lost soul. I couldn't manage to vacuum, and instead of feeling sorry for myself, I thought I'd try something that every woman knows how to do very well: grocery shopping. I'm sure I could ace that one!

# Insights and Reflections

**Listening to My Body:** One profound lesson stands out: the importance of listening to my body. On that Saturday morning drive, I felt my arm go numb. It was a subtle sign, easy to dismiss in the moment, but it was my body's way of signaling that something wasn't right. We often overlook these small cues, yet they can be crucial indicators of our health and well-being. It's taught me to be more attuned to what my body is trying to communicate, no matter how insignificant it might seem.

**The Impact of Past Health History:** My struggle with thyroid disease, diagnosed after a chance visit to Planned Parenthood, has been a key aspect of my health journey. It made me realize how past health issues can intertwine and impact our current well-being. The connection between my thyroid condition and my heart issue, Wolff-Parkinson-White syndrome, was a revelation. It's a stark reminder of how our health history can cast a long shadow, influencing our present and future health. It's made me more proactive and vigilant about my health, understanding that everything is connected.

**Finding Strength in Vulnerability and Seeking Support:** There's a moment of truth when you're standing alone, overwhelmed, and uncertain. It's a moment many can relate to - realizing that it's okay not to be able to do everything alone. This experience has taught me that reaching out for help is not a weakness but a brave step towards healing. Whether it's talking to a doctor, confiding in family, or seeking community support, embracing vulnerability is a pathway to strength. It's been a lesson in recognizing the power of seeking help and sharing my struggles, rather than facing them in solitude.

# Chapter Two

## The Day Normalcy Faded

When Laughter Stopped

~ ❖ ~
*"Tell your heart that the fear of suffering is worse
than the suffering itself."*
**—Paulo Coelho**
~ ❖ ~

I got myself together and shopped for a nice spaghetti and meatball dinner. I thought that might make things better for the family and myself. I have been on edge and very short-tempered, so it's the least I could do. It was a gorgeous, hot day, and I got into my car. I drove to a local market and parked the car. I grabbed a shopping cart and stood in the market doorway for a bit. I stood next to a large display of blueberries, and although I didn't need blueberries, something made me put them in my cart.

I was feeling uncomfortable; I felt like I had a massive pimple on my nose, and everyone was looking at me. I got a sense of being completely overwhelmed and a little confused. I was so tired of feeling this way and having these episodes of confusion interrupt my daily life. It felt like I was standing in the same spot forever, but it was probably a few minutes. The store walls started to feel like they were closing in on me, and my breathing felt tough.

I needed to start walking around, but where would I start? I knew I needed coffee, so I'd start there. I had been to this market numerous times and knew where the coffee was kept; at least, I thought I knew. "Ok, coffee, coffee, where's the coffee?" Oh no, not this again, I thought. The internal dialogue started: "What do you mean you don't know where the coffee is?" Now, I hadn't moved yet, and I started sweating profusely. I believe I was having a panic attack, and I had a sense of dread come over me.

It's incredible to me that no matter how old you are, when you don't feel well or get hurt, your first thought is, "I want my mom." At least I wanted my mom at that moment. If I wasn't a grown woman, I would have sat in a ball in the middle of the store and just started crying. I looked into the eyes of every elderly woman, and the thought crossed my mind to approach someone and ask for help. I wasn't sure what I needed help with, but I could've used someone's support.

I took a few steps towards the aisles and looked for the coffee. I must have read the list of items down each aisle five times and had no idea what I was reading. I kept saying to myself, "Come on now, just take a breath and calm down; you can figure this out; you can do this." I walked up and down the aisles feeling completely lost; the anxiety and panic intensified. A large part of me wanted to just run out of there and leave, but another part felt stubborn.

I continued to have internal arguments with myself. Everything I tried to read became a blur. I thought if I could find the coffee, I could leave. I felt silly walking around a grocery store and leaving with nothing. It's like stepping into a restaurant and using the bathroom. I must have blacked out for a moment because I don't remember purchasing anything before I left. The next thing I knew, I was back in my car.

As I pulled out of the parking lot, I was determined to go to another grocery store where I knew where all the items were. I still wasn't feeling myself, and I looked in the rear-view mirror because I swore something was wrong with my face. I arrived at the next grocery store, not far from my home. I started to take a deep breath because I was back at my old stomping ground, and it made me feel safe, like a comfortable pair of jeans.

I got out of my car, went to the second grocery store, and tried to navigate it. I was not leaving without a few items and, of course, my coffee. I can't say I remember much, but I do recall walking up and down the pasta aisle because that was a favorite of mine. I grabbed a couple of boxes of ziti, spaghetti, and sauce jars. Jarred sauce is a big no-no in my mother-in-law's house, but it does the trick in my house. I went to the milk aisle because we always need milk. I grabbed some yogurt and chocolate pudding and felt like I had accomplished what I had come to do, so I checked out and headed home.

My phone rang as I returned to my car, and my oldest daughter was on the other end. She sounded worried and annoyed. She began the conversation with, "Oh my GOD, mom, where the heck are you, and what's taking you so long?" I hadn't felt like I was out that long, but then I realized I had been out all day.

I finally reached back home, and both my girls were playing Barbies outside on the stoop with the next-door neighbor. It was a hot, beautiful day, and I couldn't wait to unpack the car and relax. I asked my youngest daughter to run inside and ask my husband to help me with the groceries. He came out to help me, and his feathers were still ruffled from earlier in the day, so he didn't say much. He emptied the car and brought everything into the kitchen. I came in right behind him, and when I walked into the kitchen, I noticed all the brown bags outlining the cabinets on the floor. I had a moment where I felt overwhelmed, like I had a tight turtleneck on. I hung my purse on the back of a chair and attempted to unpack all the groceries.

I took a visual inventory of the room and remembered seeing spaghetti and sauce peeking from the bags. The minute I noticed them, I said, "Ok, now that's spaghetti and sauce in the bag, but where do they belong, and what do I do with them?" Why am I asking myself these questions, and why don't I know their answers? All this confusion seemed very strange, but I still tried to finish what needed to get done. I turned to the fridge and recalled seeing pudding or yogurt and became confused about what compartment they belonged in. Now I'm really annoyed; what in the world is happening here?

I turned around, and my youngest daughter was standing across from me. Our eyes met, and I could feel like she was looking through me. I tried to take a deep breath and calmly ask her where my husband was. I knew I needed him immediately, but I didn't want to scare her. I said, "Sweetheart, do you know where Daddy is?" Before she could answer me, something told me, find your husband, and find him now! We lived in a small townhome, so there was only a tiny hallway separating the kitchen from the living room and a flight of stairs leading to the bedrooms, where I believed he was.

I slowly walked down the short hallway to the bottom of the staircase and felt my border collie come up from behind me. He used his snout to nudge my hand as if to say, "Hey, Mom, what's going on here?" Feeling his cold, wet nose on my fingers brought me back to the present moment. I looked down at my right arm, and my hand was pulled down almost past my knee. Oh boy, I thought, that can't be good. If I had been offered a million dollars to lift my arm at that moment, I wouldn't have been able to do it. I mumbled a few curse words and proceeded up the stairs. I have no memory of physically climbing the stairs alone; I swear a power greater than myself got me to the top.

When I reached the top of the stairs, I turned and stood in front of the bathroom door and banged on it as if my life depended on it, and it did. My husband, of course, was in the bathroom and needed his privacy, so not knowing what I wanted, he yelled back, "Uh, I'm in the bathroom, and I'm busy." He knows my voice in an emergency and must have understood because he opened the door very quickly. I don't know who looked worse, him or me. I looked at him and thought, Boy, I must look horrible because his face looked awful. I could tell by the look in his eyes that the right side of my face must have been drooping.

He put his arms out and caught me under my armpits right before my right leg gave out. The right side of my body was completely dead weight, and he had to drag my lifeless body down the rest of the hall into our bedroom. He tried hard to get me onto the bed, but it was impossible. Initially, only the right side of my body was on the bed, and the left was hanging off. He stood next to the side of the bed and pushed my other half onto the bed. I lay there, and the right arm and leg that were once dead weight automatically turned inward; my right arm and hand came up to my chin and started uncontrollably shaking. My right leg looked dislocated and curved inward towards my other leg.

I was lying on a pillow, and my head felt like it was being pulled back, and my chin was straight up in the air. I kept mumbling, "Something's wrong, call 911, something's wrong, call 911," as if he couldn't figure that out on his own. I'm sure he was saying to himself, Thanks for the heads up, Einstein.

He left the room momentarily, and the next thing I heard were loud sirens from police, ambulances, and fire trucks. I thought, wow, is this all for me? Well, it was all for me and gave me a reality check. I could hear a lot of commotion coming from outside and loud footsteps up my stairs. Our hallway was very narrow, and a standard stretcher couldn't make it. Lucky for me, they had a potato sack or hammock-looking apparatus. The paramedics came up to my room and started to test me. Ok, we all know timing is crucial during a stroke, and I was with it enough to understand he was wasting my precious time. He looked at me and said, "Ma'am." I thought, Ma'am? I'm over forty, but I'm not a ma'am yet.

He continued, "Ma'am, can you smile?" Smile? Does it look like I can smile? No, I can't friggin smile. Next question. So, he continues, "Can you squeeze my two fingers? Do you know what month we are in?" Now I'm not only having a stroke and a seizure, but I also can't smile, I can't squeeze your fingers, I have no idea what month it is, and you're wasting my time! Finally, I heard those words, "CODE STROKE, CODE STROKE." I've never been so happy to hear those words; at least now I knew I would be cared for. For the most part, I was alert and awake and remembered every detail. I had small periods that I forgot because the next thing I knew, I was in that bungee cord, hammock-looking thing, and my head was bobbing up and down while being carried down the stairs.

The paramedics got me downstairs and opened the door to my front steps. As soon as the door opened, I was surrounded by my two girls and every neighbor in the complex. I felt like I was being sent to the principal's office. I was carried down the front steps, curled up like a sack of potatoes. I couldn't see around me, but I knew my girls were watching. I tried to put myself in their shoes for a moment and asked myself, "How would I be feeling or reacting to this situation if I was watching my mother have a stroke and being placed in an ambulance?" I knew the answer, and it didn't feel very good. I was feeling anxious and scared, and I couldn't imagine what my poor girls were feeling. I tried my best to reassure them as I was being carried through the crowd that Mommy would be okay, but I didn't know if I was telling the truth. I had a lump in my throat from sadness, tears in my eyes, and an awful feeling in the pit of my stomach.

I've heard that life goes fast, but was this it? Was this the last time they would see their mom? Ugh, it all became unbearable and utterly overwhelming for me to digest. I was placed on a stretcher outside in the parking lot before I went into the ambulance. As the ambulance doors opened, everything became surreal. I was placed headfirst into the ambulance, and the doors were shut after I was inside. Everything was so cold and sterile, and I remember seeing the crisscross silver backing of the doors and speaking to God. I was very calm, and I said, "Please, GOD, please don't take me now; my babies still need me." For a moment, everything was quiet, and I was alone, or was I?

# INSIGHTS AND REFLECTIONS

**The Importance of Acknowledging and Addressing Anxiety:** As I stood in the grocery store, overwhelmed and lost in my thoughts, it was clear how profoundly anxiety can impact our daily lives. The feeling of being watched, the panic at not finding the coffee aisle, the wish for my mother's comfort—all these were signs of deep-seated anxiety taking hold. It taught me how crucial it is to recognize and address these feelings rather than brushing them aside. Dealing with anxiety is not just about managing the moment but also understanding and addressing the underlying issues.

**The Connection Between Physical Health and Emotional State:** My struggle to perform simple tasks like shopping or unpacking groceries was a stark reminder of how closely our physical health is linked to our emotional state. The confusion, the inability to remember basic things—they weren't just physical symptoms; they were manifestations of my inner turmoil. This experience showed me the importance of caring for not just the body but also the mind.

**The Power of Instinct and the Need for Support:** When I couldn't even recognize the familiar settings of my kitchen or understand where to store groceries, it was my instinct that finally kicked in, telling me to seek help. And in that critical moment, my body and mind worked together to direct me to my husband. This taught me to trust my instincts more and reinforced the importance of having a support system. It's okay to lean on others when we're not at our strongest – in fact, it's often necessary.

These insights have profoundly shaped my understanding of myself and my approach to life's challenges. They remind me of the delicate balance between our physical and emotional well-being and the power of human resilience.

# Chapter

## Three

# Unraveling the Ties

## Family, Secrets, and Redemption

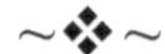

*"The way to learn whether a person is
trustworthy is to trust him."*
**—Ernest Hemingway**

*S*itting here and reminiscing about where I've been and how I got here blows me away. Not knowing exactly where to begin, in a way, I guess, is my beginning. So, as a very young child, I suffered from debilitating depression, and as the years went by, I felt that it became worse and more chronic. I felt like I was always getting by, almost like just passing a midterm with a 65. I always longed to be seen and included, but I never felt confident enough to stick my neck out for it. I remember walking through my high school hallways and feeling sadness in the pit of my stomach for being a part of the drama club. They would have tryouts and rehearsals for upcoming plays, and as much as I wanted to be included, I was petrified with absolutely no self-esteem. It was a very lonely place to be, and looking back, as uncomfortable as it was, it was comfortable and all I knew.

I would walk back and forth to school, wanting somewhere to be and someone to be with. As I walked and got closer to home, I remembered feeling like, "UGH, I'm so tired of doing the same old thing." I would get inside, drop my backpack, have a snack, and good old depression would come over. I could smell the stale smoke everywhere, as it permeated everything. I would lay on the couch and watch reruns of old sitcoms, wishing I was included in some activity after school but too depressed to want to be a part of anything. It was always this constant emotional struggle with me.

For years, we lived in my home and couldn't afford to make any renovations. We moved into my home in 1980 when I was eight years old. When my mother mopped the floors, the tiles were so old, dry, and cracked that the colors would run into each other in the water. The cabinets on the wall were made of white metal and were scattered about with no rhyme or reason. The kitchen also served as a laundry room, and the washer and dryer sat underneath the cabinets where we kept our cereal.

I remember having a rotary phone on the wall, and it made me happy when the cord was long enough to reach the dining room. After many nights of crying and arguing with my mother about how awful the house always looked, which added to my depression and constant feelings of frustration, my parents finally renovated the kitchen when I was 15. I felt like I had hit the lottery and felt proud enough to have friends over. Although the house was cosmetically in better shape, I continued to struggle with my "friend" depression.

My father chose to sleep on the couch in our living room and thought nothing about making the living room look like a bedroom. Let's say bedrooms tend to have a bedroom-type smell that we should keep out of the living room. He was a heavy smoker, so his cigarettes, ashtrays, pajamas, blankets, pillows, clothing, and shoes all took up space in our living room. He also had a recliner that he chose to eat his dinner in and left his dirty plates, cups, and soda bottles nearby. It was a recipe for, you guessed it, my old friend— depression.

My dad had a good heart, but there was no room for discussion when it came to asking him to clean up after himself or anything else for that matter. Whenever I could, I spent time with friends. Most of my neighborhood was made up of families from Cuba, so dinner at a friend's house was always an escape. Fortunately, I had a couple of good friends on my block who had a specific dinnertime and would always have room for one more. My mother was a nurse, and as a younger child, she worked 3-11 pm at the local hospital, so I rarely saw her. My aunt, uncle, and cousins were nearby, and they frequently had me over for dinner and sleepovers. Looking back, I realize my family never sat down for dinner together, and my mom would usually leave something on the stove for my dad. Leftovers were a staple in my home, as were many nights of Campbell's soup or cereal.

We shared driveways with one of my neighbors, and they had a young girl and boy who became our friends. Her dad was an incredible cook. I remember walking up her driveway. I could smell whatever was on the menu by the cooking vent on the side of her house. Her parents came from Cuba and spoke Spanish fluently. It was directly because of this neighbor that I could learn Spanish. To have dinner with them, I had to ask for whatever he was making in Spanish, or he wouldn't serve me dinner. At least that's the game we played.

I learned so much from their culture, and they became like family. I spent holidays and birthdays with them, and I even went to Florida with my girlfriend and her grandmother when we were nine years old. Looking back, my girlfriend and her mother were a massive part of my childhood, and I'll be forever grateful that they treated me like one of their own. On weekends, we would go shopping with her mom, have sleepovers, and stay up all night talking together. Her mother had a nail business out of her home, so customers were constantly coming and going, and I thoroughly enjoyed visiting with them and having good conversations.

My home was a safe place, but it was not a very happy place. My parents were more like roommates. I can't remember a time when my parents shared a bedroom, and there was always an underlying feeling of turmoil.

We moved out of the home I was born in when I was eight. I lived with my grandmother, uncle, mother, father, and two brothers at that time. My immediate family and I moved into our new home in 1980 when I was eight, and my mother went from working as a nurse at a local hospital to being a private duty nurse for a young man who was hydrocephalic and confined to his bed. His parents once had a funeral to attend, and my uncle introduced them to my mother. His parents could not leave their home without a nurse available to care for him while they were out, so my mother became his full-time nurse. I was around nine years old when my mom started working for them on weekends. She would go there in the late afternoon on a Saturday and stay until about 1:00 a.m. Back then, Fantasy Island and The Love Boat were popular on TV, and my mom and I would make Lipton soup, watch TV, and I would sit on the edge of the young boys' bed and read to him. He couldn't see or speak but would smile when I read to him.

After a couple of years working for this family, we all became very close. They had a pool in the backyard, and we spent most of our summers swimming with friends and family. We would celebrate the summer holidays and barbecue on the weekends. We would have big Italian dinners on Sundays, and they attended holidays and birthdays at our home. My father was not very involved in our lives, so this gave this young boy's father space to move in, and he became a father figure to me. He would take us to pick out our Christmas trees, and he and his wife would cook the seven fish dinners every year for Christmas Eve. They got to know some of my boyfriends and school friends over the years and were invited to any big life events. My mom was one of five sisters. They were invited to all my aunts' and uncles' celebrations throughout the years. When I got married and started a family, the wife came with my mom, and I would go shopping for the new baby, and they were both involved in planning my baby shower. As a young and innocent child, I only understood the façade that was on the surface. I enjoyed our time together and was grateful for this man, who stood up and became my father figure. With age and wisdom, I began to see what lies under the surface, and I realized that it was convenient for this man, who only had one very sick son, to wiggle himself into our lives; he was very controlling of my mother's life and created distance between my brothers and me from my father. It wasn't until many years later that I could come to terms with the truth. His wife was very laid-back and easygoing, so she didn't have difficulty standing back in the shadows, which worked well for him to control my mother's every move.

When I was 35 years old, I was pregnant with my first child; at six months pregnant, I lost my father to lymphoma. It was Thanksgiving in 2005, and my dad noticed a sore in his mouth. He went to our family dentist and asked if the sore could be an infected tooth. The dentist assured him that no teeth or gums were infected. He then reached out to our family doctor. From Thanksgiving 2005 to Christmas 2005, the sore in his mouth that was the size of an almond grew to the size of a ping pong ball and started to spread down his neck. At Christmas, the growth took over the right side of his neck and became the size of a tennis ball. After the New Year, my father couldn't put his chin to his chest because this growth was in the way. We all knew it was severe, but we didn't realize how serious till his biopsy in January of 2006. Right after the holidays, it was confirmed that he had non-Hodgkin's lymphoma.

My husband and I found out we were pregnant a couple of months later, in March, and I'm grateful that my dad and I spent some time together talking about my first child and his grandchild. That May, my dad went into remission, and for a little while, I was hopeful that he would recover. He stayed in remission till the beginning of July, and then cancer once again showed its ugly head. My husband and I celebrated our first wedding anniversary on July 17th, and I found out the next day that my dad had fallen down our flight of steps at home. My mother didn't want to ruin my anniversary, so she kept it a secret till the following day. My husband and I arrived at the hospital and heard the story of what had happened.

The evening he fell, he was walking across the hallway to the bathroom, and we assumed he felt dizzy and slipped down the flight of stairs. The first thing I noticed when I saw him in the hospital was that he looked like he was medicated. I questioned my mother as to what the doctors had given him, and she said, "Dad is not on any medication; the cancer came back, and it metastasized all over his body." All my feelings of being hopeful and dreaming of him meeting this new baby went out the door. Family and friends surrounded him for the time we had left, and I was able to spend some quality time with him before I had to say goodbye. On July 25th, my dad took his last breath, and we sent him off with all the love we had.

Once again, the couple that my mother worked for stepped up as grandparents, but deep down, it was coming from a very selfish place. He and his wife celebrated all the milestones with the new baby, and she even grew up to know them as grandma and grandpa. I was grateful after losing my father that my first child had someone to call grandpa, but unfortunately, I felt it was coming from a toxic place. Four years later, we had another little girl, and she also called them grandma and grandpa.

It wasn't until my youngest was about six years old that all the years of secrets and lies came to the surface. I had made plans with my husband and girls to visit my mother on Christmas day. She was in an assisted living home for her Parkinson's. I specifically asked that they not attend, and when we arrived, they were there. Something deep down inside me erupted and exploded, and I made a scene in front of everyone. My husband and I stormed out of the facility with our girls, and from that day forward, they never saw or spoke to any of us again. That alone showed me the truth I had refused to see for many years. Birthdays, Christmas, and anniversaries came and went—not a peep from either of them.

Part of me is resentful and hurt, but when I get upset, I remind myself of the underlying motive of having total control over my mother's life, and I feel better. After having that emotional blowout, my relationship with my mother was tattered and torn, and I felt for years that they were always a priority in my mother's life; I don't know if I'll ever completely heal from that hurt. My mom and I had much work to do to heal our relationship. They have both since passed away, and that has given me some degree of closure to the past; I'm now able to start over with my mother and heal some of those old wounds.

# INSIGHTS AND REFLECTIONS

**The Weight of Childhood Depression**: As I look back, the heaviness of childhood depression stands out starkly. It wasn't just a fleeting sadness; it was a deep, chronic condition that colored my world. I longed for inclusion, for a place in activities like the drama club, but my low self-esteem shackled me. This constant battle with depression, even amidst the mundane walk to and from school, was a silent companion that affected how I saw myself and interacted with the world.

**The Impact of My Living Environment**: The moment my parents renovated our home when I was 15 was transformative. It taught me the power of one's surroundings on mental health. This change in our home brought a sense of pride and shifted my perspective, even if it didn't fully lift the cloud of depression. It was a valuable lesson in how our environment can influence our inner state and contribute to our sense of self-worth.

**Navigating Complex Family Relationships and External Influences**: My life has been deeply affected by my family dynamics and the influence of people around us. The complicated relationship with the family my mother worked for, and their integration into our lives, was a complex interplay of emotions and control. It revealed the significant impact of external factors on our family life and personal development, teaching me about the complexities of relationships and the importance of setting boundaries for mental and emotional health.

# Chapter Four

## Finding My Voice

### From Childhood Whispers to Adult Strength

~❖~
*"Teachers open the door, but you must enter by yourself."*
**—ZEN proverb**
~❖~

*I* never realized how needy I was as a child until I became an adult. I was always the student in the back of the class, whispering to everyone around me if I did the assignment correctly, if I heard the directions correctly, or if my work looked OK. Boy, was I a pain in the ass! I didn't think much of being that way at the time, but I know now that it came from a place of always wanting to be right, wanting to be seen, and making sure I didn't screw up. It pains me to think back on my childhood because I didn't feel accepted or safe with big or small decisions in my life.

I remember being about twelve years old, and we had a pizzeria around the corner from my house. My girlfriends and I would go there on the weekends and for lunch during school. I guess I was crying out for attention, and it didn't matter who it came from or if it was negative or positive. A young man worked there, and I believe he was about twenty-seven. He would talk to me and compliment me. He made me feel special and seen, and as a twelve-year-old, I didn't care who was on the other end of the conversation, just if someone noticed me. I guess it felt wrong in a good way, but I didn't have the confidence or boundaries to stop it. Somehow, my mother found out about it and immediately confronted the gentleman. If I'm not mistaken, he was fired immediately.

As I'm typing this, I'm having difficulty because I can't come to terms with the fact that I'm speaking about myself. I went from a place of a lot of sadness and feelings of being less than.

I also had an experience with a young couple renting an apartment in our basement. They had traveled here from Cuba and just had a new baby. My mother would work long hours on the weekends, and most of the time, I was home with my dad and didn't have much to do. One Saturday evening, I knocked on the tenant's door and wanted to play with the baby. The young couple welcomed me in, and we sat and talked for a bit. The young mother decided to bathe her son and excused herself from the kitchen. Her husband and I continued to talk at the kitchen table. He would point at objects around the house and say them in Spanish, and I would translate them into English for him. We were going back and forth, and he pointed to a pair of black socks on the floor beside him. I said, "In English, we call them socks." The minute I looked back up at him, he had unzipped his pants and exposed himself to me.

I remember feeling sweaty and frozen in fear. I didn't know what to do or say, so I got up and told his wife that it was getting late and that I needed to get upstairs. I left their apartment, went up to my back door, and walked past my father in his chair in the living room. I was still in shock and speechless. I felt ashamed and didn't know where to turn for help. I kept it a secret the whole weekend, and on Sunday night, I got very upset and told my mother the entire story. Unfortunately, the situation went from bad to worse. We had to get the police involved, and I had to tell them the story in detail.

The husband worked at a local hospital, and I remember the police waiting in my driveway for him to get home after his shift. They arrested him that night. It was a very uncomfortable place for everyone, and my parents told them they had to move out immediately. Taking inventory of my childhood as a grown woman, I understand the energy I gave off as a child and the energy I attracted. It takes a lot of therapy and soul-searching to wrap your head around it. I thank God that my experiences turned out OK in the end.

Twelve years old was a pivotal year for me. I became interested in boys and had my first major crush on a boy who attended a public school in a neighboring town. My mutual girlfriend lived very close to my crush, and I spent a lot of time at her house. I was very uncomfortable in my skin, and when I heard he would be hanging out with a group of us, I was full of butterflies. I desperately wanted him to like me, and if he gave me any attention, I felt so special. There was a group of boys and girls, and we would walk around the neighborhood, try to get into a park at night, and neck in the woods. I remember feeling jealous because I found out he liked my girlfriend and his friend liked me. It seemed always to turn out that way; you always want what you can't have.

My early teenage years were full of a lot of trying to fit in and depression. High school was tough, and I felt very awkward. I was a decent student; I went to class, did my homework, and stayed after when I needed extra help. My freshman year was uneventful. My best friend was still in 8th grade, and we would go to each other's houses and have sleepovers on the weekends. Sometimes, we would take a bus to our local mall. One time, I remember meeting some young boys and exchanging phone numbers.

We ended up dating from time to time. We would spend the day with them. I remember taking a bus to their house during my sophomore year when their parents worked; we did what teenagers do best. I was nervous, scared, unprepared, and guilty. My best friend and I were always on a mission, and most of the time, we got away with a lot of trouble. One time, she came to my house, and we sat outside my bedroom window on the roof and drank vodka straight. Obviously, we didn't know what we were doing. I remember it burning so bad as it went down and thinking, if this is what being an adult is like, I'm not interested.

Summers were spent going to my mother's job, swimming in their pool, or spending the weekend in Connecticut with my girlfriend's parents. We would stay up late, eat boxes of Froot Loops, and spend every waking minute together. We were more like sisters. I can't remember a time when we weren't together. I find it funny that when you're young and best friends with someone, you think it will be like that forever, and that's not the case. When we were eight and nine years old, we couldn't imagine our reality any different from how it was. Summers seemed to last forever, and we soaked up every hot day together.

We would walk to the park during the day, run down to the cold stream, sit in it, and talk and laugh. We would ride our bikes together at night and hang out with all the neighborhood kids on our block. Our street was filled with many kids, and all the neighbors knew each other, so staying out was safe for us. My curfew was when the streetlights came on, and my best friend and I would get my portable record player and sing and dance on my porch to Grease.

Most of the time, we were young and innocent, but I liked the rebel side of her. It made my adrenaline rush, and it was exciting. When we were still in elementary school, the most exciting thing was going to the seventh and eighth-grade dances on Friday nights. Her crush went to our school, so they were always together, and I always awkwardly danced with whoever was interested. I remember the very uncomfortable way the girls would put their hands on the boys' shoulders, and the boys would hold us around our waists. It was a moment of, OK, what do I do? What should I say? When my best friend and I were together, I never felt noticed. She was always the prettier one and the one all the boys liked. It was upsetting not to feel seen. As far as I can remember, I never felt seen or worthy.

She was the one who would take cigarettes from her dad, and we felt so cool when we were smoking. As we became older teenagers, we both smoked, and I remember the first time my mother found a pack of cigarettes in my purse. Boy, was she disappointed in me! I smoked occasionally but never really enjoyed it. Once again, I thought it would help me fit in. I now know I wasn't born to fit in; I was born to stand out!

When my family and I moved from the home where I was born to the house we had owned since I was nine years old, my uncle stayed behind and lived in my childhood home by himself. We had a very close relationship, and I would spend much time with him after school and on the weekends. He never had children, so my brothers and I were like his own. He didn't take care of himself, and he suffered from diabetes. When I was about fourteen, his legs had to be amputated due to neglect from diabetes. He was confined to a wheelchair, and my oldest brother decided to move in with him and take care of his needs. I was a sophomore in high school when he passed away. I remember every detail about that night like it was yesterday. We only lived down the block from him, and I was in my bedroom with the window open. I swear to this day, I heard the paramedics say, "Grab the oxygen," and I knew at that moment he was gone. Sophomore year was probably one of the worst years of my life, and I fell into a deep depression. I attended school because I had to, but I don't have many memories of that year other than crying often and being depressed.

My mother thought therapy would benefit me, and I found a reputable social worker near my high school. I went to therapy every week, and we discussed a lot of painful memories. I put a lot of effort into healing, and I'm grateful I had the support. The rest of my high school years were much better than my sophomore year, and I was starting to turn the corner with my mood. During my junior year, the energy in the school was very easygoing, and we were all looking forward to graduating soon. Looking back on my high school years, it wasn't all bad. At the end of my junior year, a bunch of my friends were hanging out, and I was introduced to one of their mutual friends. We quickly became a couple and dated from when I was seventeen to about twenty-four years old.

Moving through teenage relationships, I encountered many highs and very lows that set the stage for my future relationships. After learning about energy and bonding with people who gave off the same vibes as myself, I now know that our bond was due to different types of traumas that we both endured as children. I learned a lot and realized I put myself in very destructive positions. After your heart is broken by your first love, there can be strong feelings of anger and rebellion. I didn't always make the best choices and said yes to men often because I didn't know how to say no.

Because I struggled with low self-esteem and confidence, I worried that saying no would make someone disapprove of me and then drop me, just like a hot pancake. I now realize that all came from a place of neediness and no self-worth, and luckily, I came out unscathed. With years of maturing, therapy, and a lot more confidence, I wish I could go back and tell her to stand up for herself and never give in to any situation that makes you uncomfortable.

There was a period between twenty-five and twenty-eight that I was partying every weekend, drinking heavily, and couldn't keep track of the men I was dating. It was a reckless time in my life, and although it wasn't productive, I'm glad I experienced it.

On October 28th, 1999, I attended a Halloween party with my best friend, and once again, I was swept off my feet by a gentleman. My love life was in a whirlwind, and things escalated very quickly. Sometimes, when you're in love, you tend to look the other way, and I do this often. Things were said and done that made me very uncomfortable, and I kept looking away and pushing them down. There were more unhappy times than happy times, and I remember taking inventory of my relationship and second-guessing it.

After about a year, we discussed marriage, and part of me felt like I was too involved to turn back. There were a bunch of red flags, and after a physical altercation, I had to come to terms with the fact that this relationship needed to come to an end. The venue was picked out, a deposit was put down, and all the invites were sent out. Family and friends were returning their RSVPs, and I had to do the unthinkable. Six weeks before the wedding, I returned the ring and called off the wedding. I had a lot of backlash to deal with, but it was well worth it. Sometimes, when you're so involved, you can't be objective about your situation. It takes a negative experience to make you realize what's best.

Calling off the wedding was one of the most challenging things I had to do, and no one could do it for me. I called friends and relatives from far and near, said the wedding was off, and returned all the gifts. Once again, I was angry and hurt and wanted nothing to do with relationships. I spent some time getting to know myself again. I got together with friends on the weekends and spent time drinking and meeting new people. We had been having fun partying on the weekends, and I was enjoying my freedom.

Being thirty and single was very difficult. I always saw myself growing up, getting married, and having a family. Canceling my wedding made me feel like all the dreams I had growing up were now squashed.

Sometimes, life gives you hardships, so you can appreciate when the good times come. After a couple of months of partying on the weekends with friends, I decided to spend time with a very close cousin of mine. We went to a bar close to home and ordered some drinks.

I noticed a good-looking gentleman sitting at the bar, and the bartender was a friend of mine. I decided to shimmy up to the crowded bar and excuse myself from being in the way of the gentleman and another customer. At first, the gentleman was very distant and cold. As I waited to be served, we struck up a conversation.

He wouldn't look my way or give me any eye contact. The conversation continued, and I noticed a large mirror behind all the liquor on the bar. I realized he had been looking at me through the mirror the whole time. When he finally looked at me, our eyes met, and we couldn't look away.

He offered to buy me a drink, and, of course, I accepted. My cousin had been waiting for me to get back with my drink, and I introduced her to the man at the bar. We all sat at the bar together and drank and chatted.

It got late, and my cousin was getting tired, so she asked me if I was ready to go. I came with her, so I felt it was best to go with her. By now, this young man and I had talked for hours, and he politely asked if he could walk me out to the car. We all stepped out, and he kissed me good night.

He had agreed to follow us to my cousin's home, and then we would get a bite to eat together. As my cousin and I were driving, I mentioned that my father had known a relative of his for many years, and we had mutual friends between us. Because of this, I felt comfortable leaving my cousin's car and getting into his car.

Our conversation was fun and easy, and we ended up at a local diner. It was three or four a.m. before I got home. The following day, he called me and left me a message on my voicemail around two p.m. I heard him speak, but I let the voicemail pick it up; I didn't want to seem too excited.

I let a couple of hours go by and called him back. We planned on going to Arthur Ave. in the Bronx for our first date. If I remember correctly, our first date was also on my grandmother's ninetieth birthday. I had to participate in her party, and he decided to pick me up from her house. I introduced him to my mother, and we left for the night.

When I got in the car, he apologized for the wet seat. He went on to tell me that his mother gave some friends of theirs a large seafood platter, and he drove his mom and dad to a local pharmacy to buy a card. He went into the pharmacy with his mother. When he came out, his father was distraught and apologized because he had to move the car out of the tow-away zone, and the fish platter was on the dashboard. When he moved the car, it all landed on my seat.

I remember sitting in the car all the way to the Bronx, and when I got out, my bottom was damp. It was a conversation starter, and it's been a long-standing joke. We arrived in the Bronx, and he picked a well-known restaurant. I don't remember what he ordered, but I got the gnocchi, and he ate all his dinner and mine. After our first date, we were inseparable. Conversations were so easy, and we laughed so hard we cried.

I was in school to learn ultrasound, and I was doing my clinical at a nearby hospital. I would finish school and head to his parents' house for dinner every night. He was between jobs and had just moved from Kansas after a divorce, so he stayed with his parents. His family and I became very close, and I enjoyed being with them all.

On the weekends, I would stay over and have a change of clothes for my clinicals on Monday morning. He worked as an auto mechanic in a family-owned business until he could figure things out. One of his best friends worked for an incredible construction company and mentioned that they might be looking to hire him.

He scheduled an interview on a Friday after the holidays and drove to Baltimore early that morning. Before the end of that evening, he had called and said he had been offered the job. There was one little problem; it was in Baltimore, and he had to be there the following Monday. We were both so excited because this was a great career, but being apart would also be very difficult.

After his interview, he came home, packed his things, and moved to Baltimore. He stayed with his best friend until I could move in with him. I was in ultrasound school to become a sonographer and graduated on May 4th. We agreed to continue our relationship long-distance, and he came home every weekend.

We would both look forward to Friday because he would drive 4 hours from Baltimore to New York and get home in the early evening. We spent the weekend with his parents, and instead of leaving on Sunday night, he got up at four a.m. on Monday morning, drove four hours, and then had a whole day of work ahead. I knew at that time that he was a keeper.

We continued our long-distance relationship from December 2003 to May of 2004. I finished my clinical in ultrasound and graduated in the first week of May. I had packed up my car and moved to Baltimore with him, and we were excited to begin our lives together. Things were challenging for a while, and we didn't have much money.

A contractor on his job was renting out the basement of a log cabin home, and it was perfect for us. He worked with his construction company, and I looked for work in ultrasound. I visited nearby hospitals to see if there were any openings for ultrasound positions. No one would give me a chance because I graduated from a different state and had no experience.

It was frustrating and disappointing, but I continued to look. I decided to look for something else while I came up with an alternate plan. I found a nearby childcare center that was hiring. Having had a lot of experience with daycare, I was hired on the spot. I worked in the three-year-old room, and I enjoyed my time there. It helped pay the bills, but it certainly wasn't where I wanted to be long-term.

We loved our new home together and had our parents visit from time to time. My husband had young children of his own, and they came from Kansas to visit during the summertime. It was a cozy cabin in the woods, and it came with everything you could want and even things you didn't.

One evening, we were outside in the backyard, a very wooded area. We opened the garage and saw a long black rope hanging in one corner of the room. He pulled on it, and it squirmed up into the ceiling; it wasn't a rope. We called his friend or landlord, and he was very nonchalant about it. He said, "Oh yeah, those are black garden snakes; they won't hurt you." After that incident, we noticed them in the garden and steered clear of them.

It wasn't long before his best friend's father was renting a two-bedroom house about 45 minutes north of where we were. He asked if we were interested, and we said absolutely. We were so excited because it was a beautiful brick home on 4 acres. We settled into our new home nicely and were even able to make some updates, such as putting in new kitchen flooring. We painted the whole house and made it our own. We loved barbecuing with friends, shopping at the outdoor mall, having an evening dinner, and discussing our future.

In January of 2005, his friend stopped by. They were chatting in the kitchen. The next thing I knew, they called me in to talk. They both took out a calendar and said, "Pick a date." I said, "Pick a date for what?" They said, "For our wedding." I guess it was sort of an informal proposal. I was in shock and didn't believe them. I thought this was a big joke.

We all talked and settled on July 17th because he had young children from a previous marriage, and they lived in Kansas. We wanted to make sure they were involved and available. I only had about six months to plan; thank God we knew what we wanted. Our timing was perfect. We had our backyard barbecue wedding on July 17th, 2005, and it was perfect. The attire was casual, and my husband wore a black T-shirt with a tuxedo printed on it, black shorts, and a pair of black high-top Converse. Everyone came in summer casual, and some brought their bathing suits. We catered to the kids with a dunk tank, bounce house, and karaoke machine; the adults had a ball. Our wedding was memorable for so many reasons, and one of them was the heat.

It was summer in Baltimore, and the night before our wedding, it poured buckets of cats and dogs. Our family and friends went out to dinner, and on our way home, we were drenched. My nerves started to get the best of me, and I was worried that my wedding would get rained out because it was planned in our backyard. The morning of my big day was overcast and foggy, with the temperature at 90 degrees and rising. The air was so thick you could cut through it with a knife, but I didn't care because it wasn't raining.

As the day moved on, I went to get my hair done, and as we left the salon, the sun came out, and it was hot and humid. When I returned from getting my hair done, my fiancé was cutting our 4 acres of grass. I was annoyed and mentioned that we were saying our vows in the next hour. My father walked me down the aisle to my husband, and there wasn't a dry eye to be seen. We had my stepchildren as our maids of honor and best men. My father-in-law had to finish my husband's vows for him because he was overcome with emotion. There was a ceremony for my stepchildren, and my husband and I gave each a ring. We said our vows before noon, and afterward, everyone jumped in the dunk tank.

Seeing the most distinguished relatives let their hair down and get dunked into the water was nice. The children jumped in the bounce house to all hours of the night, and my new husband and I sang karaoke. We had hired a barbecue catering service, and at the end of the night, we took the rest of the food to the hotel where we were staying. When we arrived at the hotel, we went to the pool, and afterward, we sat on the bed and finished off barbecue ribs. The rest of the evening's details are left to the imagination.

The next morning, we met up with family and friends near the water at Inner Harbor. My husband's children were with us, our parents, and some aunts and uncles. We shopped, went to lunch, and enjoyed everyone's company. We waited a couple of weeks before our honeymoon, and I'm so happy I did. It was nice to settle in and get organized before we left.

# INSIGHTS AND REFLECTIONS

**Seeking Validation and Attention**: Looking back, I realize I was constantly seeking validation and attention, especially in my school days. Always asking for reassurance on my work or if I'd understood things correctly, I see now that it stemmed from a deep need to be seen and to be right. This neediness, which I understand now, reflected my lack of self-esteem and confidence. It was a way for me to feel accepted and to avoid making mistakes, which I feared might make me feel even more invisible or inadequate.

**Vulnerability to Inappropriate Attention**: My interactions with older men during my childhood, like the incident at the pizzeria or with the tenant, highlight a troubling aspect of my need for attention. As a young girl, I didn't have the boundaries or the self-confidence to navigate these situations safely. This vulnerability led to experiences that were confusing and, in hindsight, deeply inappropriate. These incidents have made me realize the importance of understanding and teaching healthy boundaries and self-worth from a young age.

**Struggles with Self-Worth and Making Healthy Choices**: My teenage years were marked by attempts to fit in and a persistent struggle with depression. As I navigated the complexities of high school and early relationships, I often found myself in situations where I felt unseen or unworthy. These feelings influenced my decisions and interactions, often leading me to seek approval in unhealthy ways. As I look back, I see a pattern of behavior driven by low self-esteem and a lack of self-love, which I now recognize as crucial areas for personal growth and healing.

# Chapter
# *Five*
# Journeys of Joy and Sorrow

A Honeymoon
Shadowed by Illness

~ ❖ ~
*"We waste time looking for the perfect lover instead of creating the perfect love."*
**—Tom Robbins**
~ ❖ ~

We left for the Dominican Republic the first week in August, and it was the trip of a lifetime. We were so carefree, and it was wonderful to call him my husband. We made friends with other couples that were on their honeymoon. We all got together in the mornings for breakfast and in the evenings for dinner. There were always activities going on. We played volleyball in the pool, saw comedy shows in the evening, and had drinks at the bar all night. Traveling as husband and wife was wonderful, and we were getting used to our new roles. Our honeymoon was a blast, but we both looked forward to returning home.

We were back home in mid-August, and the summer was winding down. We started getting into our new routine as husband and wife and were happy. He went back to work, and I stayed home. As the colder weather approached, we were excited to spend our holidays together as men and wives.

We traveled back to New York for Thanksgiving. That's when we learned my father hadn't been feeling well. He was suffering from what he thought was an abscess in his mouth. He went for some testing, and we weren't sure what we were dealing with. It was a waiting game; we would know more in the next few months.

When we arrived back in Baltimore, we were looking forward to starting a family. For some couples, having a child is not so much work, but for us, it has become a job. After being married for a bit, we both realized we needed help in this area because it wasn't happening naturally. I suffered from thyroid disease; the thyroid is a master gland that controls every aspect of the body, including the hormones and reproductive areas. I was grateful that we lived in Baltimore because we were very close to Johns Hopkins, and they were a tremendous support for reproductive endocrinology. I contacted the correct department for our needs, and the doctor met with us quickly.

During our first visit, we spoke about my health and the history of my thyroid disease. We had set up another appointment for several procedures to see what we were dealing with. The procedures were quick, and there were no complications. They went through my belly button with a camera and looked at my reproductive organs. I was told that they had removed a small amount of endometriosis and that we should have success. After about three weeks, the doctor mentioned that we could resume all normal activity, and we got right to it.

I believe the doctor gave us the go-ahead in February of 2006 to start trying to conceive. In March, we decided to move back to New York after learning that my father had been diagnosed with lymphoma. I remember feeling exhausted and irritable during the move, and it was very difficult to drive moving trucks from Baltimore to New York when you're tired to begin with. When we arrived home, there was a lot to unpack and get settled. We decided to live with my in-laws for a bit and earn some money together before getting our own place. My in-laws had been in Florida when we arrived in March, so we had the house to ourselves.

Out of curiosity, I purchased a pregnancy test early one morning. My husband left for work, and I was excited to see the results. I stood in the bathroom, and I knew the drill. Five minutes felt like hours, and finally, I saw the two lines: I was pregnant! I was like a child on Christmas morning and didn't know what to do with myself. I called my mother and told her the news, and then I came up with a plan to tell my husband.

He was working about 30 minutes away from home, and I called to see if he was busy and if he could meet for coffee. He said that he was free, and I headed to his job. If I remember correctly, I showed him the pregnancy test, and he was in total disbelief. He wanted me to take a couple more, and they all confirmed the same thing: we were going to have a baby. For the next few months, we enjoyed learning and researching the baby's growth and development and dreamed about how he or she would look.

By the time May came, we received the news that my dad's cancer had gone into remission. We were all so happy and thought he was on the right track. June came and went without any real changes, and then in July, he wasn't feeling well.

I was about five months pregnant at the time, and we were getting ready to celebrate our first wedding anniversary, which was on July 17th. The two of us and my stepchildren had dinner reservations at the same place where we had our first date. The evening was beautiful, and I was grateful to spend it with my stepchildren.

The following day, I received a call from my mother that my dad had fallen down the stairs on the night of my wedding anniversary, and he was in the hospital. I was a little upset that the news was kept from me, but my mother didn't want to ruin my 1st anniversary dinner. Everyone had made plans to meet at the hospital and visit my dad. When we arrived, I saw my dad sitting on the edge of his bed. I could see that he wasn't focusing, and he looked delirious. I asked my mother what medication the doctors gave him to make him so loopy, and she said he wasn't on any medication. I realized then that things were not going in the right direction. We were told that the cancer was back, and it had most likely metastasized to the brain. It was a short period before he passed away, and family and friends all visited to say their goodbyes. I thank

God my stepchildren were visiting from out west because they got to spend time with him and create lasting memories.

A couple of days before my dad passed, we all gathered around his bedside, and he gave us all special messages. When he was speaking to my husband, he said, "Please take care of my girl for me," and there wasn't a dry eye in the room.

The night before he passed away, my mother asked my husband and me to get to the church and see if a priest was available to give my father his last rites. We knocked on the door where the priests lived, and only one priest was available. My father was born in Bratislava, and the priest who was available was leaving for his home in Bratislava in the morning. Another God Winks!! We told him the story about my dad, and he said he would come to give him his last rites. When we arrived at the hospital, the priest approached my dad and spoke to him in Slovak. Suddenly, my father started speaking back to him in Slovak. My father hadn't spoken a word of Slovak in over 30 years. The conversation didn't go very far, and he kept speaking in circles, but to hear him speak the language blew us all away. After the priest left, we all had some private time with my dad to tell him we loved him. When I was a little girl, I remember lying on his chest and feeling so safe. He would sing or hum, and I could feel the vibration of his voice. The last time I spoke to him, I laid my head on his chest and whispered, "It's ok, you can go home now; your mom is waiting for you." I want to believe I gave his spirit permission to go because the next morning, at 6 a.m., we got the call that my dad had passed away. Being almost 25 weeks pregnant and losing your dad is probably one of the hardest times I've ever had to experience.

His wake and funeral were planned, and because he served in the Navy, they had them come to drape his casket with the American flag and play Taps. The pain of losing my father while pregnant with his grandchild was indescribable. Being at his wake was somewhat of a blur. I remember mentioning to my mother that I was feeling cramping and a tightness in my abdomen. I was in my sixth month of pregnancy at the time. At seven months pregnant, I was working as a 1:1 special education aide in my local school district. When I reached the 7-month mark, I started to have Braxton Hicks' contractions throughout the school day. I left school early a handful of times, and the last time, my doctor monitored me for a couple of hours at the hospital and then put me on strict bed rest.

The night we buried my father was my first experience with a true panic attack. We all slept at my in-laws and had all come upstairs to bed. I went to the top of the staircase and asked my husband why he had turned the TV on downstairs and why the volume was so high. He turned and looked at me and said, "I used the bathroom downstairs. I never touched the TV." I guess that was my father's way of saying hello! In the middle of the night, I woke up screaming. I had a dream that there was a swarm of black ants covering my neck, and I couldn't breathe. That was probably one of the worst panic attacks I ever experienced. Everyone was trying to console me, but nothing and no one could take the pain away.

My father passed away in July of 2006, and in October, my 90-year-old grandmother passed away. I was already on bed rest, so I couldn't attend. My body and my mental health were wearing thin. I continued to have contractions from September to November, when I gave birth to my daughter. My doctor thought it was best to schedule a c-section; she was under the assumption that, due to the loss of my father, I wasn't going to be able to have a natural delivery. I remember the morning of my c-section and feeling angry and resentful. It was a cold, snowy day at the end of November, and I was disappointed with myself because of the way I was feeling. I was about to have this beautiful baby that we had waited so long for, and I was not happy. I reluctantly got to the hospital and got prepared for my c-section. I think I was angry because I didn't feel like I was given a chance to see if my body could go into labor on its own. I felt cheated and frustrated. My doctor had called me a week earlier and said, "Well, we scheduled your c-section for November 28th." I was completely caught off guard, and I believed at the time that the doctor knew best.

Looking back, I didn't feel like I had a voice or a choice. Boy, if I had known then what I know now. I kick myself when I think about it, but I'm thankful everything turned out for the best.

# Insights and Reflections

**The Importance of Emotional Support in Times of Grief and Joy**: My experiences during the early years of my marriage, particularly around the time of my honeymoon and the subsequent illness and loss of my father, taught me the crucial role of emotional support. The joy of my honeymoon, shadowed by the sorrow of my father's illness, was a stark reminder of life's fragile balance. It emphasized the need for a supportive partner, especially during times of significant life transitions. This period in my life highlighted how crucial it is to have someone by your side who understands and shares both your joys and sorrows.

**Resilience in the Face of Life's Challenges**: The journey of starting a family, coupled with the emotional turmoil of my father's illness and passing, reinforced my understanding of resilience. Despite the challenges and setbacks, such as struggling with fertility issues and the emotional distress of losing a loved one, I learned the power of perseverance. These experiences taught me that resilience isn't just about enduring hardships but also about finding ways to move forward and embrace life's joys, such as the birth of a child, even in the midst of grief.

**Navigating Personal Health and Grief Simultaneously**: My experience with trying to conceive while dealing with my father's illness and eventual passing brought to light the complex interplay between personal health and grief. Balancing the excitement of pregnancy with the profound sorrow of losing a loved one was a challenging journey. It underscored the importance of self-care and acknowledged the impact of emotional stress on physical well-being. This period taught me that attending to one's health, both mental and physical, is crucial, especially when navigating the unpredictable waves of grief and joy that life presents.

# Chapter *Six*

# Bittersweet Beginnings

## Navigating Postpartum Turmoil

~❖~
*"Don't grieve. Anything you lose*
*comes around in another form."*
**—Rumi**
~❖~

On the morning of November 28th, 2006, I gave birth to a gorgeous platinum-blonde baby girl. Every mother thinks her baby is beautiful, but my daughter looked like a porcelain doll. She was the only blonde baby in the nursery, and when anyone came to visit, they knew exactly which child was mine. She was the baby girl I waited and prayed for, and I wanted nothing to do with her. You read that right. She was a dream come true, and I was petrified to be alone with her and know that I was responsible for her. I never bonded with her, and to this day, I have a lot of shame and guilt around her birth. I didn't know any better and wasn't sure how to ask for help or where to turn. I was so ashamed of all the thoughts and feelings I was having, and I wanted to escape my life. My family was supportive, although they didn't know how to help. I found a therapist that specialized in postpartum depression, and she was very supportive.

Coming home with a new baby at the beginning of December was difficult. I was healing from a c-section and the loss of my father. I thought my depression as a child was hard. Life was about to show me a couple of lessons.

My mother would come over in the evenings, and I remember having a frog in my throat when she had to leave. I hated to be alone with this new baby, and nighttime was the worst. If anyone wanted to take my place, I would've given it to them immediately. The fear and doubt that continuously crept into my head were awful. My husband worked nights, so it was just me and the baby.

I would reluctantly get up in the middle of the night and make a bottle to feed her. I always had a lump in my throat and tears in my eyes, and I just wanted to hand her over to someone else so that I could run away from that responsibility. I had to come to terms with the way I was feeling; it brought on so much shame and disgust.

All my good friends had their children much earlier in life, so they were in a different time period with their children. I didn't feel they could relate to how I felt, and I was too ashamed to share it with anyone besides family.

I would stand beside her crib at night, play beautiful lullabies, and think, "She's so beautiful, and I waited so long to have this little girl. What is wrong with me? I don't want anything to do with her." I always felt very alone with my fear and wanted to run away. I was afraid to tell anyone how I felt, thinking they would think I was crazy. Society discusses having the blues now and then, but there is so much shame around postpartum depression and not bonding with your baby.

My days and nights with her were filled with anxiety and tears. I tried to be around friends or family as much as possible. I didn't want to be alone with her, and the thought of her being my total responsibility was so scary. I was constantly fighting depression and wanted to be a good mother. To this day, discussing this time in my life, I still feel so much shame about it. I thank God it's talked about more; hopefully, women who suffer from it get the help they need.

A lot of my depression stems from losing my father during pregnancy. I was happy that I was finally able to have this beautiful baby girl, and I was also very angry that my father was never able to meet her. I kept saying that this whole experience was bittersweet.

I believe that when GOD takes someone to heaven, he also gives life to someone else, but I never dreamed my father would be taken, and my daughter would be born.

When she was about 2 ½, we had a tag sale, and I got rid of all her baby clothes. I believe my postpartum depression lasted about two years. My husband and I felt blessed and grateful to have a beautiful, healthy baby. I was starting to feel like myself again, and I was petrified of suffering from depression if I chose to have another baby. I have gained so much knowledge about my experience of losing my father and then giving birth. Becoming a first-time mother is difficult and scary on its own; adding the loss of a parent to the mix made my life almost unbearable.

When my daughter was around three years old, I started playing around with the idea of having another child. I couldn't believe what I was thinking after suffering so much. The pain of losing my father was indescribable, but it also made me think about my daughter being an only child. My husband and I discussed the thought of something happening to us in the future and our daughter being an only child. That made me think twice, and I felt sad about the idea.

After about two years, we realized that, once again, we needed help. I contacted my surgeon at Johns Hopkins, and we made an appointment to drive there. Again, I had a bunch of testing done. The surgeon performed another laparoscopic procedure and saw that a significant growth of endometriosis completely blocked my left fallopian tube. He said he would attempt to clean out the tube and save it. If it were beyond saving, he would have to remove it altogether. I woke up with my husband beside my bed, saying, "Honey, I'm so sorry, but the surgeon did all he could to save the tube, but it had to be removed." It was a complete shock, and I felt defeated and angry.

The surgeon counseled us and said that we now had a 50% chance of conceiving. That was painful to hear, but he explained that each month, women ovulate from one ovary or the other. If we timed it right, we could be successful. The procedure was done in August, and we discovered we were pregnant in October. My period was late, so I took a test. When the test came up positive, I was beyond grateful for all we had to go through.

I was working as a school aide for the fourth grade, and we were rehearsing for a play. The staircase from our classroom to the auditorium was a couple of flights, and running up and down them all day exhausted me. After rehearsing all day, it was time for lunch. I went into the lunchroom and began to feel lightheaded and faint. I had taken the pregnancy test that morning and wasn't ready to share the news, but when I passed out, I had to share it with everyone. The principal of our school came to see if I was okay and felt it was best to send me home.

That evening, I was anticipating sharing the news with my husband. I planned to put a blue and pink bow on my belly and ask him which one he liked. When I showed him the bows and asked him to pick the one he wanted, he was a little confused. I told him we were pregnant, and he came to tears. We agreed that we would not find out the sex of the baby and save it for a surprise.

When I was about four weeks pregnant, I started to spot, and for a moment, I felt that all the hard work and planning had gone down the drain. I was so upset and contacted my OB/GYN immediately. I went in for an exam, and she performed an ultrasound. She said that what happens sometimes is called implantation, and it can cause some bleeding. She assured me that the pregnancy was fine and that it was a positive sign that the fertilized egg was implanted.

I was happy to know we were on the right track. Our first ultrasound couldn't come quickly enough. I was so anxious to see and hear the heartbeat and make sure our second child was progressing. We went to our 20-week ultrasound, and the baby was growing nicely. While we were there, the tech asked us if we wanted to know the sex. I said no, and Hubby said,

Sure, why not? I couldn't believe it; he swore we would keep it a surprise. I'm the worst when keeping secrets or waiting for something special, so I gave in. I had felt that this pregnancy was so different from my first, and I had felt up to this point that it was a boy. The ultrasound tech said it was another girl. I was a little disappointed for a moment, but when it sank in, I imagined all the special times sisters could share together and was overjoyed.

We came home that evening and told our daughter that she would be a big sister and that it was another girl. She was only 3 ½, so she didn't fully understand the concept. I enjoyed the pregnancy after feeling all the anxiety at the beginning of it. I continued to work and looked forward to having two little girls. As the months passed and I grew bigger, my doctor said, "This looks like it's going to be a big baby." Walking up and down the staircase at work in May was very difficult. This big baby was lying on my sciatic nerve, and the pain was like a lightning bolt from my lower back and down my leg. I was due in July and worked until the early part of June. Our daughter was due on July 19th.

The weekend before I thought I would give birth, my husband and I planned a nice dinner at a restaurant and a movie. My brother-in-law and sister-in-law had taken our other daughter for the weekend so we could have our last hurrah before the new baby. I was seeing a local chiropractor for sciatic nerve pain and scheduled a visit that morning before our date night. I got to the chiropractor's office around 10 a.m. and used the bathroom before adjusting. To my surprise, I saw the mucous plug had come out, and I was starting labor. My chiropractor and I laughed, and she said, "I guess there's no need to get adjusted today." I called my husband and mother and let them know what was on the agenda for the day. We were having a baby.

When I arrived home, I called my midwife and my doctor. My first pregnancy was a scheduled c-section, and this time I was going to try a natural birth. The contractions had started about an hour after I got home from the chiropractor. I was advised to stay home for as long as possible. My midwife said she would come over after a couple of hours of contractions. She came over around dinner time, and I was struggling. We thought of some different ways to make me comfortable. I had started labor at about 11:30 am on Saturday, and I wanted to stay home as long as possible.

My midwife suggested I get into the shower and let the warm water soothe my contractions. The shower was warm and comforting, but I couldn't stand there too long. I came out and dried off. As I was drying off, I felt nauseous and got sick. My midwife let us know that getting sick was a normal response and that I would be okay. I tried to walk around the apartment and took breaks on the recliner when the contractions were painful.

My mother-in-law brought some escarole and beans because Italian food helps everything. I didn't have much appetite, but I did my best and ate dinner. It was around 6/7:00, and we all agreed to head to the hospital. This is the fun part. I was having contractions four minutes apart on the way to the hospital. I kneeled in the front seat and held onto the headrest all the way there. Suddenly, my husband says, "Holy Shit." I was afraid to ask. He turns to me and says, "I missed the exit!" Oh, my goodness, I was speechless as the contractions kept coming. My husband has an odd sense of humor, so I thought he was joking. I said, "This is not the time to be kidding around." He replied, "I'm not joking." Let's say I screamed out a bunch of words that I chose not to write in my book. Thank God my midwife was following behind and knew the area. She got in front of us and led us to the hospital.

When we pulled into the hospital's parking lot, my husband helped me out of the car. A gentleman was coming from the hospital with a wheelchair for me and asked if I needed it. My husband looked at the man and said, "No, thank you, it's better if she walks?" I looked at him in disbelief and said, "Are you kidding me? He thinks he's a comedian, but his content isn't always funny. I stuck it out and made my way up to labor and delivery. On my way there, I took a couple of breaks, and the contractions became more severe.

We got to the nurse's station, and a nurse took us to a room. I got dressed in the beautiful hospital gown they gave us and settled in. I was put on the fetal monitor, and my contractions were getting more intense. At one point, a nurse told me to change my position. I stood at the foot of the bed and laid my chest over the mattress. A nurse came in and said that the baby's heart rate was low, and I needed to eat something with sugar. My husband fed me Reese's peanut butter cups. That was the first time in my life that I didn't want them. They continued to monitor the baby's heart rate and gave me some medication so I could tolerate the contractions through the night.

The next morning, my doctor and a nurse came in to examine me, and with every contraction, she did an internal exam. Let's just say by the time she was done, I didn't want anything to do with her. She discussed the plan going forward and said that I'd been laboring for 24 hours, and I was only dilated 1 cm. It was up to me to decide how much longer I would continue, but after hearing that I only dilated 1 cm after 24 hours, it didn't give me much hope. At 11:30 a.m. on Sunday, I reluctantly gave in to another c-section. Part of me felt like I failed, but the other part was exhausted.

I was taken into the O.R., and after a couple of minutes of feeling tugging and pulling, I heard the doctor say, "Whew, that's an awful lot of water." She said it covered the O.R. floor. My husband and I eagerly waited to hear our daughter cry and learn how much she weighed. We listened to the beautiful sound of her crying and asked what her weight was. The doctor said, "She's 9lbs 7oz and 21 inches long." All the 3–6-month clothing would be useless, and I thought she was big enough to start kindergarten immediately. We learned that having a c-section was the best route after she was born. My doctor came to us and said, "The umbilical cord was wrapped around her neck, and every time I had a contraction, it would get tight around her neck and cause her heart rate to slow down." I thank God that I listened to my body and intuition, and my daughter was born healthy. My pregnancy and delivery were like night and day with my second child. I find it interesting how much our emotional and mental health contribute to the upbringing of our children. My energy was in such a positive place, and even though the process was painful, I found that raising my second daughter was a breeze.

I believe there are times in our lives when we all experience triggers. I was never aware of these triggers in the past or throughout my early teenage years. When I was about 18 years old, I was watching a talk show with the topic being trauma within the family. It affected me to the point that it was deeply disturbing. Moments like this came up sporadically, and I began to pay attention to them. After suffering from debilitating depression for years without a real reason, I wondered why my reaction to this show was out of the ordinary. Was this the answer? Did something like this happen to me? If it did, when did it happen? Why did it happen? Who did it happen to? I had so many questions and no answers.

I realized I had always been empathetic, but this seemed different. I had been with my best friend that day. We had been friends since we were eight, so she knew everything about me. We dissected different situations, and deep down, I understood where all these feelings came from. Growing up in a home where I lived with my parents, brothers, uncle, and grandmother wasn't always easy or comfortable. My brothers and I were left in my uncle's care most of the time, and I recall some questionable behavior from him at times. I don't have many memories of being a very young girl, but around the age of 7 or 8 years old, there were times when I felt very uncomfortable.

I discussed the show with my mom, and she tried to be as supportive as possible. In an awkward way, this revelation I was having was both upsetting and refreshing, all bundled up in one. For years, my depression was just a part of my everyday life. It weighed me down like a heavy blanket, and there wasn't much to fix it. I went from therapist to therapist and tried different antidepressants until I found one that worked. I became very angry with myself and my life. Initially, I felt that if I agreed to take medication, it would turn me into a zombie or change my personality. I remember crying in a psychiatrist's office and feeling like everyone except me was on the same page. That was a tough place to be stuck in.

I decided to enter an outpatient program from 9-5, five days a week, to seek answers to all the questions I had about my childhood. The therapeutic program was intensive, and I learned much more about my childhood. Some things I discovered were eye-opening, and others were alarming. I finally confirmed that I had suffered, and it was at the hands of my uncle. We sat in groups and shared our stories of difficult life situations and depression, and some even discussed feelings of suicide.

I recalled a time when I was a very young child, and my uncle was looking after us. My brothers and I would come home from school, and he would be waiting for us. As a child, I felt that my uncle regularly replaced my parents. He treated me as one of his own because he was never married and had no children. He was there for us after school, served us dinner, and usually got me ready for bed.

Getting me ready for bed sometimes meant bathing me. I don't remember anything in detail, but I have flashbacks of times when I felt funny. He always pretended that he couldn't find the soap under the water, and when he found it, he pretended it was a fish that had gotten away, and I would laugh.

I also remember an oversized green and purple towel and him wrapping me up in it. I didn't think much of those experiences then, but as I grew older and looked back on my life and my feelings of sadness, I realized that it was all funny behavior between a young girl and her uncle. I remember feeling weird when I would sit on his chair or lay with him on the couch and watch baseball, but as a small child, I didn't understand why. I mentioned all this to my mother recently, and she was never aware that he was bathing me. I had assumed that she had asked him to and that she had known all along.

# INSIGHTS AND REFLECTIONS

**Postpartum Depression and the Struggle with Motherhood**: The birth of my daughter revealed a profound and painful truth about postpartum depression. Despite the joy and fulfillment most associate with motherhood, my experience was overshadowed by fear, anxiety, and a lack of connection with my newborn. This phase was riddled with guilt and shame, as I grappled with feelings of detachment and an overwhelming sense of inadequacy. It was a period marked by the struggle to bond with my child, compounded by the grief of losing my father. This chapter of my life underscores the complex emotions surrounding motherhood and the importance of addressing mental health issues like postpartum depression.

**The Impact of Personal Loss on Parenting**: My father's illness and passing during my pregnancy and postpartum period significantly impacted my emotional state and ability to fully embrace motherhood. The bittersweet mix of welcoming a new life while grieving another was a profound challenge. This experience highlighted how deeply personal loss can affect new parents, intertwining joy with sorrow. It was a stark reminder of how life's pivotal moments can be interlaced with pain and joy, significantly influencing one's parenting journey.

**Facing the Stigma Around Mental Health**: During this tumultuous period, I confronted the societal stigma surrounding mental health, especially in the context of motherhood. The overwhelming pressure to conform to the idealized image of a happy and nurturing mother made it difficult to seek help or even admit my struggles with postpartum depression. This experience illuminated the critical need for open conversations about mental health, particularly for new mothers grappling with similar challenges. It highlighted the importance of support systems and professional help in navigating the complexities of mental and emotional health after childbirth.

# Chapter Seven

# Unraveling Shadows

## Confronting a Painful Past

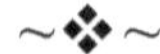

*"It's not what happens to you, but*
*how you react to it that matters."*
**—Epictetus**

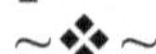

My uncle passed away when I was fifteen, and his death magnified the severity of my feelings. I was a sophomore when he passed, and I questioned my connection with him. It was upsetting to feel that a relative I loved and trusted could hurt me and cause so much confusion in my life. I was angry that I felt such sadness at losing someone who had caused me so much turmoil. How could I love and care about someone I was supposed to dislike?

I knew our relationship was very close and losing him felt like losing more than just an uncle. I always knew that my relationship with my uncle was a little uncomfortable, but I never really understood why.

During my time in the program, we had intense group therapy. I recall one session where I reacted very emotionally to someone else's story of inappropriate behavior by a relative. It wasn't until that moment that I realized how much other people's stories impacted me. A counselor took me aside and asked me what was upsetting me. I wasn't sure, but I dug deep into my emotions. The psychologists worked with me, and we delved into some very raw emotions.

During that session, I learned I had suppressed feelings about my uncle. The empathy I felt for the young lady sharing her story brought up emotions related to my situation. I sat curled up in a ball, rocking and crying in my chair. I was slowly uncovering my memories, and it felt like I was living in a nightmare. The counselors and I explored the history of my childhood, and they asked if I had ever felt that anyone had been inappropriate with me. I remembered certain situations of unacceptable behavior, and flashbacks have surfaced over the years. All these memories surfaced when I was about 18 or 19 years old. As painful as it all was, it was eye-opening to understand why I had suffered from such debilitating depression, a sense of hopelessness, and low self-esteem throughout my life.

After learning about my situation, I went through a period of anger and depression. I was in denial, and because I couldn't remember too many details, I always questioned the actual situation. Since learning about this, my life has had many ups and downs.

My brothers and I spent a lot of our childhood with my uncle. In many ways, he took on the roles of a parent, sitter, and friend. I poured my whole heart and soul into our relationship. I have fond memories of staying up late at night with him. We watched Christmas shows together and The Wizard of Oz every year. He was our caretaker and entertainment wrapped in one. We visited amusement parks, and Sunday mornings were reserved for trips to the toy store.

After learning about the history of my situation, I went through periods of anger and resentment. I struggled with feelings of trust and love for someone who had hurt me. The pain and hurt have affected every aspect of my life. As a young girl, I was very quiet and shy. As I got a little older, I never felt seen or heard. During elementary school, I tried to find out where I belonged and who my friends were.

As a young girl, I suppressed the situation, so sometimes I didn't understand my reactions to certain situations in life. Ever since I can remember, I suffered from depression, and I was never truly happy with my life. I never felt attractive or believed that anything I had to say was of any importance. Just writing this and revisiting my past brings up a lot of emotions and reminds me that I came from a place filled with a lot of sadness.

I realize now that I was a needy child, always seeking love and validation. Whenever I was attracted to a boy, I was the one chasing him. I never felt attractive or worthy enough to be wanted by someone else. I came from a place of neediness and longing to belong. I now understand that the energy I carried with me is what ultimately attracted me. I never walked with confidence and lacked self-esteem. I believed that's who I was, and I never thought anything in my life would change that. Most of the boys I liked were not interested in me, and things didn't change much for me when I entered high school.

The first two years of high school, I was very depressed and simply did what I had to do to get by. Then came the summer of my junior year, and it was the first time I felt seen and acknowledged. I had some friends from school whom I hung out with regularly, and I was introduced to one of my friend's brothers. After several evenings of getting together as a group, we planned to meet for the Fourth of July fireworks. The fireworks went off, and so did our relationship. We spent every waking minute together, and we shared a strong chemistry. He was a sophomore in college, so he had to leave in September.

We maintained a long-distance relationship on and off for about seven years, but eventually we grew apart and chose different paths. I knew I would eventually want to marry and have children, and he didn't want any of that. I was heartbroken and angry. I wasn't sure what to do with myself, so I got involved with drinking, partying, and dating several men at a time. I attached myself to others who were broken to feel like I belonged, but I realized I attracted what I believed was my self-worth. My self-worth was minimal, and after struggling for many years and learning about the situation I had suffered at the hands of my uncle, it brought all my feelings of self-doubt and depression to the surface.

I can say that after learning about someone I loved so dearly who hurt me as a child, I questioned my life and existence. I thought, 'Why would a relative that I loved, trusted, and respected do the ultimate betrayal and hurt me as a child?' That situation set me up for years of having no self-worth and questioning my purpose on this earth.

When I contemplated sharing this book and my life story, I wasn't sure where to begin. I experienced so many health issues. I was always in the hospital with abdominal pain and was examined by several medical specialists to rule out ulcers, Crohn's disease, appendicitis, ovarian cysts, and gastrointestinal issues. I felt I could talk about overcoming health struggles and feelings of despair, but I didn't know how to give my story a strong foundation. After years of soul-searching and speaking with like-minded people, I had found the answer.

The trajectory of my life happened the way it did due to the situation I suffered as a child. I started out very early with low self-esteem, not feeling heard, seen, or valued. For a long time, I accepted that that was just how my life was supposed to be, and that's who I was.

As an adult, after learning about my situation, I also discovered that any situation endured as a child resurfaces itself as other ailments. I feel that the only time I felt acknowledged was when I was sick, and whether I knew it or not, that's what was happening. I also think that emotional and physical situations get stuck in some regions of the body and manifest themselves as other problems. Most of my complaints stemmed from my reproductive organs.

I had several ruptured ovarian cysts as a teenager, and for years, I was doubled over in pain, and no one had any answers. There were multiple times I would be rushed to the hospital writhing in pain, and when I arrived, my blood levels would be checked for appendicitis. On one occasion, I was prepped for appendix surgery, and they canceled at the last minute because my blood levels were normal. One time, a doctor pulled my mother aside and said that maybe I just needed some therapy. I had been in and out of therapy for years, and I knew when I was suffering from mental health or physical health problems.

Fast forward to trying to start a family and finding out I suffered from endometriosis; my research taught me that endometriosis cannot be seen on an ultrasound, CT scan, or MRI. It can only be diagnosed during a procedure where the doctor can visualize it.

After moving from Westchester, NY, to multiple apartments in Duchess County, NY, we moved into a beautiful townhome in a gated community. We were so excited to start a new chapter. The girls had so many new friends to ride bikes with, and all the neighbors were friendly. It was the summer of 2016, and the moving truck had pulled up in front. The men were bringing furniture in, and I was doubled over in pain. Somehow, I got through the day and managed to hold out till they left. I laid on the couch and told my husband I needed to get checked out at an urgent care facility nearby.

He drove me to the closest one, and I was immediately told it was appendicitis, and I was sent to the hospital. This is where it gets good (insert sarcasm). The girls were still in school, and we had to leave them with a neighbor. My husband and I headed down to Westchester, NY, because I felt if I needed surgery, I knew the positive reputation of Westchester hospitals. I went to the ER, and they did several labs, tests, and procedures that were humiliating. I was sent home with an antibiotic and told to wait until after the weekend. The doctor said if the medication didn't help throughout the weekend, to call him on Monday morning, and he would personally remove my appendix. I didn't make it through the weekend. I called the hospital; they contacted my doctor, and he told me to come to the ER, and they would admit me.

I arrived at the hospital on a Saturday, and I was admitted immediately. Sunday morning came, and I was prepped for an appendectomy. My husband was on his way, so my mother was with me. After surgery, I was told that my surgeon was a general surgeon, and his intentions were to do an appendectomy and close me up. During the surgery, he had to consult with my mother, so he left the OR and took my mother aside. He said he had found a mass on the right portion of my colon, and he didn't know what it was, but it was abnormal. Because he was a general surgeon, he did not have the expertise to remove a mass on my colon, and he also didn't have any other surgeons available on a Sunday afternoon. He suggested that he finish my appendectomy and that I contact a colon surgeon as soon as possible.

I slowly recovered from my appendectomy and did my research on a colon surgeon in my area. I found a surgeon I felt very comfortable with, and he assured me that I would be in good hands no matter what he found. In the meantime, I feared that I might have colon cancer. I did a lot of crying and worrying while I was healing. After about 6 weeks of recovery, I was scheduled for my colon surgery. My doctor removed the right portion of my colon, 10 inches of intestine, and I had a resection of the intestine that was removed. That recovery was challenging, no pun intended. I couldn't leave the house because everything I ate or drank went through me. I lost a lot of weight, and it wasn't easy to regain my energy. I was told the good news and the bad news. The good news was I didn't have colon cancer, and the bad news was I had Stage 4 endometriosis, and it was everywhere.

My colon surgeon said that he was not an expert in reproductive organs, but he knew enough to say that endometriosis was growing in my ovaries, uterus, fallopian tubes, and rectum. He referred me to a reproductive endocrinologist, and that was the next step on my journey.

My mother and I met with a reproductive endocrinologist, and he said that from looking at the surgery that was performed previously, endometriosis had grown all over my reproductive organs like poison ivy. He informed me that our ovaries produce a hormone called estrogen, and endometriosis feeds on estrogen and continues to grow. To stop the growth of my endometriosis, we had to get rid of the culprit, and that was my ovaries. I knew enough about the reproductive system that once the ovaries are removed, the body goes into menopause. I saw the effects of menopause on my mother years ago. She suffered from unbearable hot flashes, insomnia, and mood swings. As women, we complain every month when we get our periods, but I can say that after going into menopause myself, I'd rather have my period.

We scheduled surgery for the removal of my ovaries to stop the growth of my Stage 4 endometriosis. I had mixed emotions about the surgery. I believe I started to struggle with endometriosis as a young teenager, and it just went undiagnosed for many years. I had multiple experiences with ruptured ovarian cysts. Sometimes I would be doubled over in pain, and my mother would rush me to the hospital; by the time I got there, the pain was gone, and everyone thought I was losing my mind.

A couple of years before my endometriosis was diagnosed, I would have episodes of trying to use the bathroom, and I constantly flipped from severe diarrhea to constipation. I recall one episode when my girls were very young. I had used the bathroom and was suffering so much that I started to black out. I called out for my oldest daughter, who was five then, and told her to run next door to our neighbor. We lived in a garden apartment, so neighbors were one door over. Thank God my neighbor was home, and she was a nurse. Talk about feeling totally humiliated. My neighbor came over and sat on the edge of my tub while I was on the toilet; she held me in case I passed out, and she suggested we call an ambulance, and we did. I arrived at the hospital, I was examined, and once again, the same story as usual, they found nothing. Endometriosis is difficult to diagnose, and I didn't know anything about it while I was growing up.

The morning of my surgery, I arrived at the hospital very early and got prepped. I met with the surgeon, who reviewed all the surgery details with my husband and me. I don't believe surgery took too long, and I woke up in the recovery room. After the anesthesia wore off, the hot flashes started immediately. HOLY SMOKES was the ride of my life. My ovaries were out and not producing estrogen for the growth of endometriosis, but now I had another battle to overcome—menopause.

Menopause moved in and brought all her ugly baggage. The baggage included severe hot flashes that made me feel dizzy and agitated and left a trail of anxiety-ridden emotions. Trying to sleep at night was a total joke; the insomnia was enough to put me over the edge. The mood swings felt left out, so she moved in, and she was a challenge! Oh, my goodness, I thought PMS was hard. Once a woman's body is in menopause, it depletes the hormones estrogen, testosterone, and progesterone. Loss of estrogen causes beautiful, youthful porcelain skin to crease and wrinkle. Loss of progesterone makes sleeping difficult, and a decrease in testosterone causes low energy. Well, let's say I suffered from all the above, and it was a complete shock to my system.

When I returned for my post-op, my surgeon mentioned that during the removal of my ovaries, he looked at my uterus and noticed that, due to the endometriosis and scar tissue, my uterus had completely adhered to my abdominal c-section scar. His exact words were, 'I would only remove your uterus if you started bleeding, which would indicate that you probably have uterine cancer.' He went on to say that my uterus was so severely covered with scar tissue that removing it from my abdomen would take a highly skilled doctor. He compared it to cutting through a spider web or chewing bubble gum. My body had been through so many surgeries in such a short time. The thought of having my uterus removed was daunting. I don't remember precisely the period between the removal of my ovaries and the removal of my uterus, which was a complete hysterectomy.

One thing about me is that I love to research. I started researching doctors who specialized in endometriosis and came across a highly skilled surgeon in Manhattan. I made the initial phone call and scheduled a time to see him. My husband and I collected all my previous health records and headed to Manhattan. The office was very professional, and the surgeon said he could help me. There was one problem: they didn't accept insurance. Well, this surgery would've cost us hundreds of thousands of dollars. We went back and forth with out-of-network benefits, and in the end, it still would've been an enormous amount of money. I felt a little defeated, but I have faith and perseverance that there will be an answer.

My husband's boss knew about my health struggles, and they were talking one day on the phone while I was in the car. His boss had mentioned that he had recently had his hip replaced and had his surgery in Connecticut. I don't know why I never thought of Connecticut, probably because we weren't far from New York City and most major hospitals are located there. The best hospital in Connecticut is Yelp, so that was my next adventure.

I contacted YALE Hospital in Connecticut and spoke to the OB/GYN Department secretary. I related my story to a nurse who wrote down my health history and directed me to the correct surgeon. My husband and I met with the surgeon, and we discussed my endometriosis. We went to great lengths about suffering with pain on my left side, my appendectomy, and seeing a colon surgeon who removed the right portion of my colon and 10 inches of intestine. The surgeon said they would use the Da Vinci robot for my hysterectomy. My uterus was completely adhered to my prior c-section incision, and using the robot was the safest approach.

The night before my surgery, my husband and I stayed in a hotel right next to the hospital. We had to be at the hospital at 6 a.m. the following day. We arrived at the hospital in the morning, and I spoke with my surgeon, met with the anesthesiologist, and was prepped for surgery. This was going to be the last leg of my journey with stage 4 endometriosis, so I was eager to get it taken care of. When I was wheeled into the OR, I remember feeling so overwhelmed and anxious. I had to slide off the stretcher onto an odd-looking table with stirrups. I suddenly became very emotional, and the team of doctors and I said a prayer before I was put to sleep.

I believe the whole surgery took about 6 hours, and I don't recall a lot that took place afterward. The morning after my surgery, I was told I could get up and walk on the unit. I stood up and felt very stiff, but I was determined to walk. I held onto my IV pole and walked alongside a nurse all the way around the unit floor.

It wasn't easy getting used to my new normal. I was 46 years old, and I was put into medically induced menopause. I always thought not having to deal with a monthly period would be great, but boy, was I wrong. Soon enough, I was introduced to hot flashes, insomnia, weight gain, and mood swings, and when my period took off, so did my libido. I love my husband so much, and we have a terrific marriage. It isn't easy to have feelings for someone and have the rug pulled out from under your feet when it comes to intimacy. I learned that the loss of my reproductive organs made me suffer another loss of feeling numb with any sensation or urgency for a physical connection. I find it interesting how we usually correlate loss with a person or pet. One of my losses was the intimate connection with my husband, and it's painful to grieve.

Back in 2011, I noticed a hard lump in my right breast, and I reached out to my breast surgeon. She did all the scans necessary and found a benign mass in my right breast. I called her one day and said, 'I realize that the mass is benign, but if it were in your body or your child's body, what would you do?' Immediately, she said, 'I would get it taken out.' So that's what we did. I had it removed and never thought about it again until going into menopause. The thing with menopause and hormone treatment is if you are at high risk for cancer, the estrogen that you are given can feed the cancer. I'm very in tune with my body, and I practice self-breast exams regularly.

Towards the end of 2018, I came across a lump in my left breast and contacted my breast surgeon. She performed a mammogram and ultrasound and called me three days before Christmas and said, 'I'm sorry to give you this news, but we found cancer.' She went on to say, 'I know this sounds crazy, but do yourself a favor and try to enjoy your holidays and your family. You are in the best hands, and we will get you the best care possible.' I tried hard not to come to pieces and stayed as strong as possible for my girls.

During the Christmas break, many close girlfriends were having a Christmas get-together. I wasn't feeling very festive with the recent news I was given, but I pushed myself to go. Before I arrived, I promised myself I wouldn't discuss the news I had received. All the ladies were so happy to see me, and I was glad I showed up. We didn't see each other often, so celebrating the holidays together was wonderful. We started with appetizers and drinks. Everyone was talking, laughing, and having such a great time. My girlfriend, who was hosting the party, began setting the dinner table, and we all sat down to eat. We were in a giddy mood, and I was happy. I sat next to some friends who were discussing their yearly mammograms, and I thought to myself, 'Oh boy, this is not the topic I was interested in.' I tried my best to stay strong and not get upset. I had a glass of wine, and that gave my tears permission to flow easily down my cheeks. I could see the concern on everyone's face, and I was upset with myself for caving in."

Some of the ladies came into the kitchen to comfort me and ask why I was upset. I started by telling them that I recently had a mammogram and an ultrasound. My doctor called me a couple of days ago and said that dreadful word. I went on to tell them that she promised I was in good hands and to try and enjoy my Christmas.

One of the ladies at the party overheard my conversation and told me about her experience with breast cancer. She reassured me that the technology is so advanced and that if it's at an early stage, I would be fine. Everyone did their best to make light of a touchy subject. My girlfriend, who was hosting the party, started to discuss that she worked in a therapist's office, and a gentleman known as a divine healer rents space there. She said, 'You absolutely must make an appointment with him. He has testimonies from all over the world of diseases and sicknesses that he's cured.

She gave me his contact information, and I scheduled an appointment as soon as possible. I arrived at the office to meet with this divine healer and waited to be called in. He met me in the waiting room, and we entered his office together. I sat down on the couch and made myself comfortable. He introduced himself and asked me what brought me to him and what he could do for me. I went on to tell him that I recently had a mammogram, and I was informed that the radiologist saw evidence of cancer. I also mentioned I was scheduled for a biopsy the following week, and my girlfriend, who works in this office, recommended that I come to see him.

He started off by asking me some medical questions and asked me to point with two fingers to show him the mass on my breast. He informed me that he was doing what he called a visual face map. I didn't understand the concept, but I had faith and trusted that he knew what he was doing. He asked me to sit in a chair, and then he sat beside me, face to face. At first, I was a little uncomfortable, but within seconds, I relaxed.

I could feel his energy change, and he went into a trance. He began breathing fast, then slowly, making odd sounds and forcing his breath out. My body began to tingle, and I became completely overcome with emotions. I wasn't sure what was happening, but I started crying and hyperventilating. He said, 'Congratulations, you just experienced your first miracle.' I could not describe what happened with my body or in my head. Before this experience, the mass in my breast was rock hard, like a crater or fossil. Afterward, he said, 'Feel the mass in your breast.' Again, I broke down because there was no sign of a mass. My breast was as pillowy and soft as a baby's bottom.

I hugged him, cried some more, and said, 'I cannot believe that I can say with conviction that I am cancer-free.' There was no doubt in my mind that I was okay. I walked out of there like I was walking on air. When I arrived home, I told my husband there was nothing to worry about; I was going to be fine. He said, 'I'd love to believe you, but I'll believe it when I see it.' A couple of days later, I had my biopsy, and my surgeon said she would call me with the results immediately. I feel like every time I have a medical procedure, it falls on a Thursday or Friday, and I must wait for the dreaded weekend for the results. We waited all weekend in anticipation, and I got the call on Tuesday morning.

My surgeon and radiologist got on the phone to deliver the best news possible. She said, 'Nancy, we don't know what you did or how you did it, but there is absolutely no sign of Cancer.' I sat there in disbelief and speechless for a moment, and then I got my composure. I said, 'You're never going to believe this.' I continued to tell her about my experience with the divine healer, and she said, 'I believe you 100%.' We both shed some tears, and she confirmed what I already knew. I experienced a miracle.

# INSIGHTS & REFLECTIONS

**The Complexities of Emotion in Abusive Relationships**: Reflecting on my relationship with my uncle, I realize the complexity of emotions involved in abuse, especially by a trusted family member. As a child, my bond with my uncle was one of love and trust, but as I grew older, I began to recognize the discomfort and confusion that stemmed from his inappropriate behavior. This duality of emotions – love for a family member and the pain from the betrayal of trust – created an inner conflict. It's a stark reminder of how abuse, especially within the family, can lead to a tangled web of emotions, making it difficult for survivors to reconcile their feelings.

**Uncovering Repressed Memories and Their Impact**: The process of therapy helped me uncover repressed memories of my uncle's inappropriate behavior. These revelations were both painful and enlightening, providing context for my long-standing depression and low self-esteem. Understanding the root of these feelings was crucial to my healing journey. It highlights the significance of addressing past traumas to understand and heal from chronic mental health issues. The experience underscores the importance of professional help in dealing with complex emotions and memories.

**Navigating the Aftermath of Discovery**: After acknowledging the abuse, I experienced a tumultuous mix of anger, denial, and depression. This emotional turmoil was exacerbated by my struggle to recall specific details, which led to self-doubt about my experiences. The journey through these emotions was a rollercoaster, impacting various aspects of my life, including my relationships and self-perception. This phase of my life underscores the challenges survivors face in reconciling with their past and the long-term effects of childhood abuse on mental health and self-worth. It also emphasizes the importance of a supportive environment and professional guidance in navigating these complex emotions.

# Chapter *Eight*

# Resilience in the Face of Adversity

## Confronting Breast Cancer

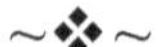

*"We are healed of a suffering only by experiencing it in full."*
**—Marcel Post**

In between having my ovaries removed in 2016, I was put on hormone replacement therapy for my hot flashes and insomnia. After my breast cancer scare at the end of 2018, my doctors recommended that I come off hormones and try something else. When you get that close to a cancer diagnosis and you're able to dodge the bullet, you choose to do anything in your power to stay safe.

I was grateful to God that I received a miracle, and I took that and ran with it. Within the following weeks, I thought to myself, I really need to come off this hormone replacement therapy, but I feared dealing with the awful hot flashes and insomnia. I was in touch with my OB/GYN and expressed my concerns. He put me on his schedule for a consultation, and within a couple of weeks, I met with him. I was excited to discuss some alternative solutions to overcoming the not-so-pleasant effects of menopause. My doctor had told me about a medication that was sold as an antidepressant but also treated hot flashes due to menopause.

I thought I hit the lotto. A medication that helps with my depression and treats hot flashes signs me up. He gave me some information and said that usually, patients start on a very low dosage and slowly increase the milligrams. I was told if I stayed on a low dosage for too long, the medication wouldn't be that potent, and I could have breakthrough hot flashes. I believe I started at 37.5 mg in February of 2019. I quickly went from 37.5 to 75. And then to 150.

In April 2019, I noticed subtle changes in my fine motor skills. Everyday tasks that we take for granted, I couldn't do anymore. We all assume that brushing our teeth and drying our hair will always be easy, but when they're taken away, we realize they are gifts. I found out after suffering from my stroke that with this medication being titrated, your blood pressure needs to be monitored for hypertension. I never had a problem with my blood pressure before my stroke or afterward. The medication was directly linked to my episode of severe hypertension, and it could've been avoided. Late April is when things became difficult, and that was when I jumped from 75 mg to 150 mg. Towards the end of May, I lost peripheral sight in my right eye, and June 2nd was my stroke.

Looking back on my medical history, it was a very long and painful journey, but I wouldn't change a thing. Each struggle was designed only for me, and every detail makes me unique. It's incredible how you can change how you see and feel about something with a small mental shift. It wasn't until I experienced my stroke that I was able to see and feel things differently. I always had the victim mentality: "Poor me. Why me?"

When God brings you so close to death, it makes you realize how fragile your life really is. Now, my mindset and internal dialogue are, 'If HE can bring me to it, HE will bring me through it.' I no longer have the victim mentality, and within every negative experience in my life, I choose to find one positive. Sometimes you win, and sometimes you learn. Either way, it builds character and makes you stronger for the next hurdle.

Speaking of hurdles, I want to discuss another hurdle that I feel I jumped with flying colors. God held my hand in the past, and I knew He would never let me down. It was November 2021, and I was going in for a routine mammogram and ultrasound. Since I am high-risk, I frequently do self-breast exams, and I thank God that I do. I had come across something that felt odd a couple of months before and tried to ignore it, but it kept haunting me.

When I went in for my exams, I brought it to the attention of the sonographer, mammogram tech, and radiologist. The sonographer was performing the ultrasound and looked at me and said, 'I don't see anything on the screen, so I wouldn't worry about it.' The mammography didn't pick up anything, either. The ultrasound tech said, 'I'll see if the radiologist is available to examine you and redo the ultrasound.' The radiologist came into the room, and I pointed to the mass in my right breast. She said, 'I feel what you're talking about, but I don't see it on the screen.' Before I got dressed, the radiologist mentioned that if I was still concerned, I should get in touch with my breast surgeon. I thanked her for her support and left the office.

From time to time, I would do a self-breast exam and get worried about the mass that I felt. I kept remembering what the sonographer, mammogram tech, and radiologist said, but something didn't feel right. I went back and forth in my head and said, 'Well, everyone said not to worry, so I'm just going to let it go,' but I couldn't. My gut feelings and intuition kept telling me to call my breast surgeon. I let it stir inside me until late January 2022, and I caved. I called my surgeon, and I told her office what I had experienced. Her secretary said, 'Well, we can schedule you for a clinical exam with the doctor.' I made an appointment and felt better about my decision.

I figured if my breast surgeon said I was fine, then I would leave it alone. On the day of my appointment, I was nervous and anxious to be examined. I waited in the waiting room until I was called. When I got into the exam room, the nurse told me to take my shirt and bra off and put on a gown. I put on the gown, sat down, and waited for the doctor.

My breast surgeon and I have known each other for over 10 years, so when she saw me, she said, "What's going on?" I explained that I had all the ultrasounds and mammograms back in November, and I wasn't comfortable with the end results. I removed the gown and she had me put my arms out, put them on my hips, and then relax. She asked what breast I felt the mass in, and I told her the right. She examined my left breast and said it was normal. When she examined my right breast, she immediately said, "I don't like it." I said, "Exactly, I don't like it either." She went on to say I wanted an MRI done. I asked, "When?" and she said, "Tomorrow."

When things like this happen, I get what I call the truth tingles. Anytime I have difficulty hearing the truth about something, my feet and toes tingle. Well, let's say they were tingling. I left the office with a frog in my throat and knew deep down that it wasn't going to be good.

I was scheduled for the MRI the next day, and it was given with and without contrast so they could see the fluid run through my breast. I don't remember too much detail about the MRI, but soon after, I was called back for a biopsy. The doctor said they saw a mass that they were concerned about, and I was scheduled for an MRI-guided biopsy.

Before arriving for the biopsy procedure, I knew in my gut that it was cancer. I was prepared with an IV, and they laid me face down on the MRI table. My surgeon and radiologist entered the MRI room and began the biopsy. My breast was marked at the area of the mass, and it was very important that I not move a finger. I felt the prick of the Novocain enter my breast, and I did my best not to wince. Once my breast was numb, the radiologist went into the breast with a device that I didn't want to look at. I was told the biopsy would make some loud noises, but it was very important that I not move an inch during the procedure. I felt a lot of pressure in my breast, but no pain.

After the procedure, the nurse bandaged me up, and I drove home. On my way home, I felt a tinge of pain in my breast while I was driving. I tried to rub my breast gently, and when I pulled my hand up out of my shirt, it was covered with blood. For a moment, I was in shock, but I continued driving.

When I arrived home, I changed out of my clothes into some comfortable sweatpants and a sweatshirt, and I noticed that I had bled through the bandages, and I was still bleeding.

I have a history of breast biopsies, and I knew this wasn't the norm. I thought it was best to notify my doctor, so I gave her a call. She said I could come back to the hospital, but all they would do was rebandage it and apply pressure. She mentioned that if my husband applied some strong pressure with his hands, it should stop, and if it didn't, get in touch with her again. Eventually, the bleeding stopped, and I was able to get some sleep. The area they biopsied was bruised and sore, and I was careful with lifting anything for a couple of days.

I believe it was a Tuesday afternoon after my biopsy. My youngest daughter and I stopped by a local Panera Bread to get something to eat. We ordered our food and sat down to eat. My phone rang, and time stood still. I didn't want to answer it in front of my daughter, but I was also eager to hear the results. I answered the phone, and the radiologist said, "Hello, Mrs. Spano." I said, "Yes, this is Mrs. Spano." If I could've run away at that moment, I would've been anywhere but there. She went on to say, "Mrs. Spano, we received the results from your biopsy, and I'm sorry to have to tell you the results are malignant; you have breast cancer." As I'm typing this, I'm feeling a little sick to my stomach, just like I did on that day.

By the way, that day was March 25th, 2022, and every 25th of the month is the anniversary of my dad's passing. He passed away on July 25th, 2006, so I know he was with me and had my back. The radiologist wasn't sure I heard her because I didn't react. My intuition knew it was malignant all along, so she just confirmed what I already knew. I said, "Yes, I'm here, and I heard you; thank you for the call." I was so calm, and I did my best to not get upset. I didn't want to upset my daughter, and I wasn't prepared to cry while I was driving home.

I told my daughter I had to make a quick call to Dad and that I would be right outside for 2 minutes. I called my husband, and he said he was in a meeting with his boss. I interrupted and said, "This is important, and I need to talk to you now." I went on to say, "OK, now I don't want you to get upset, but I just received the results of my biopsy, and the mass is malignant, I have breast cancer." He replied, "Wait, what? What do you mean? Why are you so calm?" I said, "We got this! I went on to say, "There is no doubt in my mind that I will be fine. God didn't take me from a stroke, so he's not about to take me from breast cancer. I also believed throughout this journey that I was so diligent with my self-exams at home that the cancer was caught so early, and I would be fine.

I went back into Panera Bread, and my daughter and I headed home. My husband and I spoke in detail that night, and my surgeon and radiologist scheduled a consultation later in the week to discuss treatment.

Later that week, we met with my cancer team. The surgeon and radiologist discussed some options with us, and the only option I could agree with was a bilateral mastectomy. Some women choose to have a lumpectomy and radiation, but I couldn't imagine willingly going in for radiation on a weekly basis and suffering burns to my breast. I also didn't feel comfortable knowing that radiation is not 100% effective and has no guarantee of killing every cancer cell. My agreement was to do a bilateral mastectomy, and we all agreed. My diagnosis was in March, and the surgery was scheduled for May 10th. My husband and I left there nervous and scared, but also with faith that God would watch over us.

The next couple of weeks were very emotional, and I was preparing myself mentally and physically for major surgery. We hadn't told our girls, and I wasn't sure how to approach them. I had presurgical bloodwork and EKGs, among many appointments with my surgeon to discuss post-op care.

One evening, I approached my husband and said, "I can't keep secrets from the girls, and I'm sure they sense something is wrong." I decided to gather everyone and let them know what had been happening. I asked them both to come into our room and sit on our bed. I felt sick to my stomach, having to tell them, and put myself in their shoes. If my mother told me when I was a young girl that she had breast cancer, I wondered how I would feel.

They both sat on our bed, and I began by saying, "You both know mommy has been having tests done and her yearly mammogram, right?" They said, "Yes." I continued, "Well, I thought I felt something in my right breast, and I went to my surgeon to get it checked out." My youngest blurted out, "Do you have cancer?" With a lump in my throat, I replied, "Yes." My oldest daughter got up and walked out of the room. I followed her and reassured them both that I would be OK. I told them I was sure that things would be fine because I knew that the cancer was at a very early stage and the mastectomy would remove anything that was growing.

May 10th arrived, the day of my mastectomy. To this day, I'm still amazed by GOD's grace. When I was 18, I got a memorial tattoo on my bikini line in memory of my uncle, the one who had abused me. His memorial date happened to be on May 10th. I bring this up because I am now 50 years old and have had this tattoo since I was 18. Over the years, I underwent painful laser treatments to remove it. After spending an enormous amount of time and money, my breast surgeon said, "I must cut right through your tattoo for a certain part of the surgery." I remember saying to myself, "Thank You, GOD!!!" After all those years of regretting my decision at 18 and getting ready for breast surgery and a new beginning, this was just what I needed.

The surgery began around 6 a.m. and lasted 7 to 8 hours. I woke up in my room feeling like the heat was turned up to a blowtorch. An inflatable blanket was laid on top of me, and heat was being forced out all around my body. It was used to increase blood flow after surgery. A nurse said it could be removed shortly, and she took it off. I was relieved that the surgery was over, but I knew I had a long road ahead of me in my recovery.

Drains were in both breasts and on either side of my hips. Some parts of my recovery in the hospital are foggy, and I don't remember if I was able to use the bathroom the night of surgery or if it was the next day. When I could get out of bed and walk to the bathroom, I had to use the call bell for a nurse. I hate asking for help, and I always try to see how far I can go on my own. The first couple of times, I used the call bell, but not long after, I was doing it on my own.

My surgeon prescribed morphine for pain, but I only depended on it for the first two days. After that, I relied on Tylenol and Motrin. My surgery was on a Tuesday, and I returned home on Saturday. I give credit to my husband's ex-wife for informing me about being entitled to a nurse when I was home. I didn't realize cancer patients were entitled to that, and I was so grateful. My nurse showed up on Monday morning and came twice a week. We developed a wonderful friendship, and she always kept my worries at bay until I could ask my surgeon my questions.

I had to drain the tubing coming out of my breasts and keep a log of how much came out daily. This was a tedious and difficult task, especially when you're in pain and exhausted. During these tough times, you feel like it's never going to end, but I maintained a positive attitude and regained a little more strength every day. I celebrated small wins like being able to shower and stand up long enough to make some hot soup. I couldn't sleep in my bed for about 3 weeks, so I slept in a recliner. After sleeping in a recliner, you truly appreciate your bed again.

Showering was incredibly difficult because I couldn't bend down, raise my hands over my head, and soap up between tubing while avoiding removing stitches. By the time I finished showering, I felt like I had run a marathon. My husband and I would follow a procedure to create an antibacterial space, drain the tubing, and measure the collected liquid. I often sat in the recliner and drifted off to sleep.

I spent a lot of time resting and watching TV. One of my best friends visited the following weekend and brought an incredible vase of flowers. When life gets tough, it's comforting to know which friends you can count on.

My visiting nurse was with me until my post-op appointment with my surgeon. When I met with my surgeon after about 2 ½ weeks, she removed my drains and said I was healing very well. I was very meticulous about taking care of my sutures and drains, and I didn't suffer any infections. The visiting nurse and I developed a special bond, and it was difficult to say goodbye.

I had such a positive mindset, and I was anxious to heal. Before my cancer diagnosis, I would spin 2-3 times weekly, and I was looking forward to getting back to my routine. I received the clearance to exercise. I began to feel healthy again and was on the road to recovery. My cancer was found behind the right nipple, so unfortunately, I lost both nipples to my breast. I don't think women realize how emotionally attached to our nipples we are until we are at the point of possibly losing them. When you see your body look a certain way for 50 years, and then a cancer diagnosis changes it, it takes a lot of getting used to. My daughters used to try and make light of the situation and say, "Mom, your boobs look like the wafer inside an Oreo cookie."

My family was so supportive throughout this journey, and my daughters helped me with every small, difficult task. I feel we take so much for granted in our lives until it's taken from us. I couldn't bend over to tie my shoes or pick things up, and my girls were there for every little thing. Sometimes, I would get emotional and start to pity myself, and my oldest would say, "Mom, it's OK, don't be upset. You just had major surgery."

# Insights and Reflections

**Navigating the Challenge of Medication and Its Consequences**: My journey with breast cancer was further complicated by the medication I was on for hormone replacement therapy. Initially, it seemed like a blessing, addressing both my depression and menopause symptoms. However, the escalation of the medication's dosage led to significant health issues, including a stroke. This experience highlights the delicate balance of medication management, particularly in complex health scenarios like mine. It underscores the importance of monitoring and adjusting medication, understanding its potential risks, and being vigilant about changes in one's health.

**The Power of Intuition and Self-Advocacy**: Despite reassurances from medical professionals, I trusted my intuition about the mass in my breast. This decision to advocate for myself, even when medical tests initially showed no cause for concern, was crucial. It was my self-examination and insistence on further evaluation that led to the discovery and treatment of my breast cancer. This aspect of my journey underscores the importance of being attuned to one's body and advocating for oneself in the healthcare system. It's a powerful reminder that patients often need to persist in their pursuit of answers, especially when their intuition tells them something is not right.

**Resilience in the Face of Overwhelming Challenges**: Facing a cancer diagnosis and undergoing a bilateral mastectomy was an incredibly daunting experience. It brought emotional turmoil, physical challenges, and the necessity to adapt to significant changes in my body. Yet, throughout this journey, I found strength in a positive mindset, the support of my family, and a deep faith. My approach to cancer, focusing on the positive in every negative situation and believing in my ability to overcome, highlights the power of resilience and a positive outlook. This resilience not only helped me cope with the immediate challenges of surgery and recovery but also aided in adapting to the new reality of my body and life post-cancer.

# Chapter
## *Nine*

# From Recovery to Revelation

## A Journey of Faith and Fulfillment

~❖~
*"You cannot protect yourself from sadness without protecting yourself from happiness."*
**—Jonathan Safran Foer**
~❖~

In February 2023, I had my last and final surgery to reconstruct my nipples and put the finishing touches on my breasts and abdomen. I'm cancer-free and ready to conquer any obstacle that comes my way.

As I sit here and contemplate the good, the bad, and the ugly, I'm grateful for the adversity in my life, the people who crossed my path to teach me lessons, the ones who left, and most of all, the ones who stayed through it all.

Throughout my life, I always had a strong faith that I was meant for more. I knew deep down that being resilient was my superpower, and having a positive mindset would prove to be successful. Back in 2021, I was scrolling through Instagram on a Sunday night when I came across a gentleman that I had previously heard share his story on the CLUBHOUSE app. There was an option to speak with him live, and I don't know what came over me, but I clicked on it. I introduced myself and was shocked that I had the nerve to speak with him. I mentioned that I heard him share his story on the CLUBHOUSE app, and he acknowledged that. We started a great conversation; he asked me my name and where I was from. We talked a little about his story, and I shared a piece of mine. I told him that I had suffered a stroke and how I felt it was an awakening to this part of my life. He had just been introduced to a young lady on CLUBHOUSE, and they were collaborating to create a faith-based group for speakers. I never considered myself a speaker, but I realized that I was an expert on overcoming adversity, having a positive mindset, and realizing that with faith, you can jump over any hurdle. He said that ZOOM classes were scheduled to start in a couple of weeks and asked if I was interested. I wasn't sure what I was getting myself into, but that kept my interest. We exchanged each other's contact information and said goodbye.

A couple of days later, I went to the website that he mentioned, and I signed up for the classes. The first night we were scheduled to meet, I was so excited and a little nervous. I love meeting new people, hearing new stories, and sharing my story. There was a small group of us, and we all introduced ourselves. It was nice to meet people from all over the United States and listen to the hurdles that they overcame. I met teachers, businessmen, and talented musicians. The group was diverse, and I was really enjoying myself. We met weekly for about 6 weeks. We had workbooks and homework, and we also had partners to hold us accountable. I looked forward to the class every week, and I learned a lot about myself.

This speaking group had started to feel like family, and I was upset at the thought of having to say goodbye. Everyone was able to share what they walked away with, and when it came to me, I said, "I've always preached to my girls to find their passion and purpose, but I never knew mine." I went on to say that I knew I loved people, listening to their stories and sharing mine, but I took that for granted. I never realized that what I had done all my life had been my purpose all along. It took so much adversity, pain, and struggle to open my eyes and bring me to that exact moment. I will be forever grateful to those two human beings and God's grace to help me find my purpose.

The faith-based speaking group that I now consider family is EMBRACE YOUR AMBITION (EYA). I was scheduled to meet them all in Colorado last year, but at the last minute, I was recovering from my mastectomy, and I couldn't make it happen. I was heartbroken and devastated. I believe we make plans, and God laughs. I couldn't see the road ahead of me, but he knew. A year later, I again signed up for the EYA conference, but this time, I decided to take my husband with me, and I thank God I did. We have always had God as the center of our marriage and our family, so this wasn't new territory.

We weren't sure what to expect, and what we witnessed changed our marriage and our lives. I can only imagine the analogy of a woman's experience with childbirth. Every experience is different, and every woman is different, and if you're not a woman, no matter how much someone goes into detail, there's no possible way to grasp the concept. We witnessed the Holy Spirit entering and exiting each one of us. We stood, strangers, arm-in-arm, while Marcus Black prayed over the room, and it left everyone crying and embracing each other like we were family. It's an emotion I wish I could put into a bottle and keep forever.

We made lasting relationships that we will treasure forever, and we also networked with like-minded people. I look forward to working with many of them on some level. EYA had a speaker who was a gentleman with a black belt in karate. He demonstrated an exercise with a piece of wood. We were told to write on one side a limiting belief we had and, on the other, something we would be capable of doing without that limiting belief. Then we had to break through it, literally and physically. Mine was that fear would hold me back from obtaining my highest potential.

My highest potential and goal are to travel to 3rd world countries and speak to women and children about overcoming situations as a child. I want to use my expertise to teach women how to use their strength through adversity. They will be able to propel themselves forward so they can reach their goals and dreams. After the exercise, a speaker sitting in the audience tapped me on the shoulder and said, "Connect with me before the end of the conference. I travel to 3rd world countries, and I can help you." I couldn't believe what I was hearing. As I've said before, another God Wink.

As far as I'm concerned, there are no accidents. God places people on our path to guide us on our journey, and everyone He's placed on my path, I'm so grateful for. The young lady and I connected before the weekend was over, and when we arrived home, I scheduled a call with her. She has a ministry retreat for women and couples. My husband and I would like to attend the couples retreat when the time is right, and I will have the honor of fulfilling my dream by speaking with women and children. My journey has had many ups and downs, and many times I wanted to throw in the towel. When I was experiencing anger, sadness, or depression, I felt as if it would never end. Sometimes, we can't see our way out when we are so deep in our misery. As human beings, we feel that in order to get answers, we should always be looking, searching, and doing, but it's when we become still that God speaks to us and prepares us for what lies ahead on our journey. I'm grateful for all the people who stood beside me and had my back, and I'm also grateful for the ones who didn't believe in me; they gave me the motivation to keep going.

As the ambulance doors opened, everything became surreal. I was placed headfirst into the ambulance, and the doors were shut after I was inside. Everything was so cold and sterile, and I remember seeing the crisscross silver backing of the doors and speaking to God. I was very calm, and I said, "Please, GOD, please don't take me now; my babies still need me." For a moment, everything was quiet, and I was alone, or was I?

The energy shifted, and the paramedics gave off an urgent vibe. My blood pressure at the time was 200/110. Instead of getting myself worked up and frightened, I felt a peace come over me like a warm white blanket. It was at that moment that my deceased father stood behind me, and I could feel his embrace on my shoulders. He whispered, "It's all going to be ok." God then said, "If I let you stay, you will agree to walk in your purpose and share your story." I wasn't alone; I'm never alone, and I will continue to keep my promise.

# INSIGHTS AND REFLECTIONS

**Discovering Purpose Through Adversity**: My journey through breast cancer, stroke, and subsequent recovery led me to a profound realization of my life's purpose. Joining the faith-based speaking group, EMBRACE YOUR AMBITION (EYA), was pivotal. It allowed me to connect with others who had overcome their struggles and share my experiences. This experience made me realize that my lifelong inclination towards empathy, resilience, and storytelling was not just a part of who I am but my actual purpose. The adversity I faced was not just a series of unfortunate events; it was a path leading me to this revelation and to embrace my role as an inspiration and guide for others.

**Transformative Power of Faith and Community**: Attending the EYA conference with my husband marked a significant turning point in our lives and marriage. The experience of feeling the Holy Spirit and the deep connections formed with others at the conference were transformative. It reinforced the idea that faith and community are powerful forces that can bring about profound personal change. The conference wasn't just an event but a spiritual journey that deepened my faith and solidified my commitment to helping others. It also opened doors to new opportunities, aligning with my newfound purpose of speaking to women and children in third-world countries about overcoming adversity.

**Commitment to Fulfilling a Promise to God**: The moment of my stroke, when I felt an overwhelming sense of peace and heard reassuring words from my late father and God, was a turning point. It wasn't just a close brush with death; it was a covenant with God. In that moment of vulnerability and near loss, I made a promise to walk in my purpose and share my story. This commitment has become a guiding principle in my life. It's not just about survival; it's about living with intention, sharing my experiences to inspire and support others, and fulfilling a divine mandate that was clarified in my most vulnerable moment. This promise keeps me focused on my path and fuels my passion to make a meaningful impact in the world.

# Chapter Ten

# Embracing Resilience

## Navigating Life's Tides with Hope and Purpose

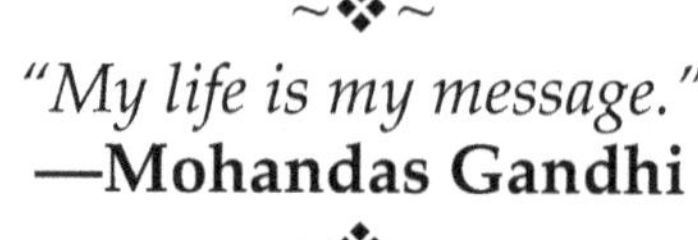

~❖~
*"My life is my message."*
**—Mohandas Gandhi**
~❖~

As I sit down to reflect on the journey that has been my life, I am struck by the intricate tapestry of experiences, each thread representing a challenge, a lesson, or a triumph. From battling health issues to facing personal adversities, every twist and turn has contributed to the person I am today. This final chapter is not just a summary of my story; it's an invitation to you, the reader, to see your challenges through a lens of resilience and purpose.

My life has been a testament to the power of resilience. Confronting breast cancer, surviving a stroke, and battling through the physical and emotional toll of these experiences taught me the profound strength inherent in the human spirit. These weren't just health crises but turning-point events that reshaped my understanding of life and my capacity to endure and thrive. Your struggles, whatever they may be, are also opportunities for growth. They are not just obstacles but catalysts for developing an inner strength you might never have known existed. Remember, resilience isn't about not falling; it's about learning how to rise every time you fall.

Throughout my journey, I discovered that pain and challenges are often the most potent teachers. Joining the EMBRACE YOUR AMBITION (EYA) group and engaging in faith-based activities didn't just offer support; they unveiled my true purpose. I realized that all my experiences, as harrowing as they were, equipped me to inspire and guide others. You, too, have a unique story and experiences that can empower not just you but others around you. Your pain can turn into your purpose if you're willing to explore what your experiences are teaching you. Your trials could be shaping you into a role you've never imagined – one where your story becomes a beacon of hope for others.

The transformative power of faith and community has been a recurring theme throughout my life. Whether it was feeling the embrace of the Holy Spirit at the EYA conference or finding solace in the shared experiences of others, I learned that we're never truly alone in our struggles. Your faith, whatever form it may take, and your community, however you define it, are invaluable sources of strength and comfort. Lean on them, contribute to them, and watch how they can transform not just your life but also the lives of those you touch.

One of the most profound lessons I learned was the power of transforming personal pain into advocacy. My health battles led me to speak to women and children in third-world countries, sharing my story to inspire and educate. This wasn't just about healing myself; it was about using my experiences to ignite change and bring hope to others. In your life, consider how your experiences could help others. Can your story educate, inspire, or advocate for change? Never underestimate the impact you can make when you turn your pain into a platform for helping others.

My life has also been an excursion into self-discovery. Through each health scare and personal challenge, I uncovered layers of myself that I never knew existed. I discovered strengths I didn't know I had and passions that lay dormant. Your journey, too, is about discovering who you are and what you're capable of. It's a continuous process of learning, growing, and evolving. Embrace it with an open heart and a curious mind.

Gratitude and grace have been my companions on this journey. Despite the pain and challenges, I found countless reasons to be grateful. This mindset shift was crucial. It helped me focus on the positives, no matter how small, and maintain a sense of balance and peace through the toughest times. As you navigate your challenges, try to find moments of gratitude. They can be as simple as a kind word from a friend or a beautiful sunrise. These moments of gratitude can be powerful anchors in the stormiest seas of life.

Finally, this journey has been about embracing the promise of tomorrow. Despite the uncertainty and fear, I learned to look forward with hope. Each challenge was not just a hurdle but a stepping stone to a brighter future. Your journey, too, is filled with promise. No matter how dark some days may seem, remember that there is always hope. There is always a chance for a new beginning, a new adventure, and a new story to write.

With all its highs and lows, my journey has been a profound lesson in resilience, purpose, faith, and the transformative power of our experiences. As you continue on your path, remember that your challenges shape you into the person you are meant to be. Embrace them, learn from them, and let them guide you to your own unique purpose. Remember, your story is not just about surviving; it's about thriving and leaving a legacy of strength and hope for others to follow.

# THANK YOU...

To everyone who has taken a moment to walk with me through the pages of my life, my heart is full of appreciation. Sharing my story with you has been a profound expression of trust and vulnerability, and your openness to receive it is a gift beyond measure.

My journey, with its highs and lows, has been a testament to the unyielding power of hope, the undeniable strength of courage, and the transformative magic of gratitude. As you hold these words, know that they are more than just sentences on a page; they are beacons of light intended to illuminate your path.

May they serve as gentle reminders that, no matter the darkness, there is always a spark of hope waiting to be ignited. Let these words of love and inspiration guide you, comfort you, and remind you of the boundless courage that resides within you.

*"Every sunrise brings a new opportunity to shine, even after the darkest nights. Embrace the light within you."*

*"Strength isn't just about enduring; it's about how gracefully you rise after a fall. Remember, every setback is a setup for a comeback."*

*"Gratitude transforms what we have into enough and more. Count your blessings and watch your life begin to overflow with abundance."*

*"The courage to continue is what turns ordinary into extraordinary. Keep pushing forward; your breakthrough is just around the corner."*

*"Hope is the heartbeat of the soul. Keep it alive, and it will carry you forward through anything."*

*"In the tapestry of life, every challenge is a thread of strength, woven together to create a masterpiece called 'You'."*

*"Miracles happen to those who believe in the power of hope. Keep believing; your miracle is on its way."*

*"Your story isn't over yet; it's just getting to the good part. Keep turning the pages and embrace the journey ahead."*

*"Let gratitude be your compass and love your pathway. Together, they lead to a life of fulfillment and joy."*

*"The strongest people aren't those who show strength in front of us, but those who win battles we know nothing about. Keep fighting; you're stronger than you think."*

*"Embrace your struggles like the stars embrace the sky; even in darkness, they shine bright."*

*"Faith is seeing light with your heart when all your eyes see is darkness. Keep faith close, and you'll never walk alone."*

*"Courage doesn't always roar. Sometimes, it's the quiet voice at the end of the day whispering, 'I will try again tomorrow.'"*

*"Hope is the only thing stronger than fear. Let it be your guide, not your shadow."*

*"Remember, the most beautiful rainbows come from the rainiest days. Keep looking for your rainbow."*

*"In the symphony of life, gratitude is the music that plays in harmony with our soul. Play it loud, play it proud."*

*"You are a lighthouse in someone's storm. Never underestimate the impact of your light."*

*"To find courage, sometimes all you need to do is take the next small step. Progress, not perfection, is what truly matters."*

*"Gratitude turns what we have into enough. Start each day with a thankful heart and watch your world change."*

*"Never lose hope. Just when the caterpillar thought the world was over, it became a butterfly. Your transformation is coming."*

# ACKNOWLEDGEMENTS

First and foremost, I must thank God for giving me this life and His gift disguised as my stroke. If not for a second chance, none of this would be possible. I'm grateful for the trials and tribulations that have brought me to this moment. I believe all roads lead to our purpose, and it is up to us to choose them wisely.

**David Lloyd Strauss — Author Coach and Editor**

Before I acknowledge the most important people in my life, I want to thank my writing coach and editor, David Lloyd Strauss. Our paths crossed in a serendipitous manner through Clubhouse, a platform that has been instrumental in the journey of this book. David's expertise, support, and encouragement have been pivotal. When I found myself in turmoil while completing this book, he was there. David didn't just offer guidance; he took the scattered pieces of my experiences and helped me mold them into a narrative that I hope will inspire and resonate with many. His insight and dedication have been a beacon of light in this process, making what seemed like an insurmountable task not just possible but a reality.

**Marcus Black and Ashlee Fay (EYA)**

Thank you to Clubhouse; if not for the app, I wouldn't have the ability to connect and network with the most amazing professional entrepreneurs, speakers, and authors. A big shout out to Marcus Black and Ashlee Fay (EYA). Marcus and Ashlee were two of the initial pieces of this thing called life that set me on my way to finding my purpose. I will be forever thankful to you both. I'm thankful for all the members of EYA for having each other's backs and holding each other's hearts; you are all my brothers and sisters.

**Amberly Lago and Samantha Harris**

Years before I ever dreamed any of this was possible, I connected with an incredible woman who gave me tremendous inspiration with her story. I want to thank Amberly Lago for defining true resilience and becoming someone I can call my friend. Because I connected with wonderful people like Amberly, I was also able to connect with a fellow warrior and breast cancer survivor, Samantha Harris. Samantha continuously uses her platform to help women obtain a healthy lifestyle and heal from the inside out. I'm thankful for being in her circle and grateful that someone with her status has been authentic and compassionate towards the breast cancer community.

**Dr. Ranjana Chaterji — Surgeon**

Thank you to my breast surgeon, Dr. Ranjana Chaterji, for cheering me on through breast cancer, having my back, and my boobs. I also want to thank my brilliant plastic surgeon, Dr. Julie Vasile. She has pieced me together in more ways than one.

**Tom and Tiffany Coverly — Dear Friends**

They say the best friendships are made in the hallway. I don't know who "they" are, but they are right. I want to show my appreciation for Tom Coverly and his wife, Tiffany. My husband and Tom met in the hallway at a conference. Tom is a gifted gentleman who tours the country to spread kindness to teenagers and puts smiles on their faces with magic tricks. Tom & Tiffany have continuously expressed their love and support for my husband and me, and we are proud to call them friends.

**Amanda Yoa. Mike C-Roc Ciorrocco. Princeton Clark.**

To my fellow girlfriend and warrior, Amanda Yoa, for welcoming me on her podcast and creating a comfortable place to share my story. Through hundreds of conversations and hours on Clubhouse, I've also had the honor of sharing my story in multiple rooms because of the generous people who have opened the floor and handed over the mic. I want to thank Mike C-Roc Ciorrocco for holding some kick-ass rooms where I was able to speak and network with like-minded individuals. I'm grateful to Princeton Clark for helping me understand my trauma, dissecting it with me, and teaching me about using your pain to leverage your life.

**My husband, Rob. My children, Ava and Abigail.**

I want to thank my husband for supporting me emotionally and financially so I can continue to work on becoming the best speaker and author. A big shout out to my girls, Ava and Abigail. My goals and dreams have taken a lot of time away from them, and I'm grateful that they've been so supportive and understanding that I'm working so hard for all of us. I'm grateful for my stepchildren and step grandson's continuous support and encouragement throughout this process.

**Mom & Dad**

To my mom, I'm grateful for your words of wisdom and for always being a constant source of support. Without my father guiding me figuratively and spiritually, I would've thrown in the towel years ago. Anytime I experienced feelings of doubt, I could count on my father to send me God Winks.

**Grace & James Spano**

"I would like to thank my in-laws, Grace and James Spano, who are now in their early 90s. For over 20 years, they've welcomed me into their home and treated me like one of their own. I will be forever grateful for the love they've shown to their granddaughters, the countless nights of babysitting, and the most incredible homemade Italian spaghetti and meatballs every Sunday afternoon. I will cherish the memories of holiday meals and the cookbook collection of all Nona's special recipes."

## Stephanie Arnold

To Stephanie Arnold, for being the very first person to plant the seed for this dream of mine to flourish and grow. Stephanie listened to me share my story with a vision and intent that she felt before anyone else could.

# ABOUT THE AUTHOR

Nancy Spano's life is a testament to the extraordinary power of resilience and the human spirit's capacity to overcome. As a devoted wife, nurturing mother, and compassionate daughter, Nancy's journey through life's rollercoaster has been nothing short of inspirational.

Since her early fascination with the complexities of the human psyche, Nancy has been on a relentless quest to understand and unravel the mysteries of the mind. Her academic pursuit in psychology wasn't just a path of learning; it was a deeply personal journey fueled by her own experiences and a burning desire to make sense of life's intricate challenges. Each hurdle she encountered, from battling childhood depression to facing physical health scares like breast cancer, didn't just test her; it sculpted her into a beacon of hope and strength.

Nancy's life story, as reflected in her writings, isn't merely a narrative of events; it's a saga of transformation and triumph. It's a profound reminder to all of us that the darkest moments of our lives can be the birthplace of our greatest victories. When she faced a stroke, it wasn't just a challenge; it was an awakening, a pivotal moment that reshaped her entire outlook on life and her role in it.

Her mission now is one of empowerment and inspiration. Nancy dedicates herself to lifting other women, guiding them through their unique journeys with wisdom gleaned from her own. She doesn't just coach; she transforms lives, encouraging women to rise above their challenges and to advocate for themselves and their dreams. Nancy teaches that within every hardship lies a seed of opportunity, a chance to grow stronger, wiser, and more fulfilled.

Her message is a clarion call to all who face adversity: Embrace your journey with all its storms and sunshine. Through her voice, Nancy imparts a powerful truth: Life's toughest battles can lead to its most beautiful chapters. She stands as a living example that even in the midst of turmoil, there is hope, and with resilience and faith, every challenge can be a stepping stone to a life of purpose and joy.

Nancy's story is an invitation to all: Rise above, find your strength, and embark on a journey of self-discovery and empowerment. Let her life be a reminder that no matter the odds, every one of us can be a beacon of resilience, a source of inspiration, in this beautifully complex tapestry called life.

# CONNECT WITH NANCY

**Speaking. Podcasts. Coaching. Interviews.**

If you've been inspired by Nancy's story and are looking for a voice of resilience, hope, and empowerment for your next event, podcast, coaching session, or interview, she would be honored to connect with you.

Nancy's experiences have not only shaped her into a beacon of light for those navigating through their own challenges but have also equipped her with insights that inspire and transform lives.

To discuss speaking engagements, podcast appearances, coaching opportunities, or interviews, please reach out to spanonancy@gmail.com.

Nancy looks forward to the possibility of sharing her story and insights with your audience, offering encouragement, and fostering a community of courage and hope.

www.ingramcontent.com/pod-product-compliance
Lightning Source LLC
Chambersburg PA
CBHW040809120726
48005CB00012B/1352